It's All About Love:
The Story of Randall Hayes Russ

It's All About Love: The Story of Randall Hayes Russ

Robert (Opey) Russ
Robin Lindenmeier

iUniverse, Inc.
New York Lincoln Shanghai

It's All About Love: The Story of Randall Hayes Russ

iUniverse books may be ordered through booksellers or by contacting:

iUniverse
2021 Pine Lake Road, Suite 100
Lincoln, NE 68512
www.iuniverse.com
1-800-Authors (1-800-288-4677)

Because of the dynamic nature of the Internet, any Web addresses or links contained in this book may have changed since publication and may no longer be valid.

The views expressed in this work are solely those of the author and do not necessarily reflect the views of the publisher, and the publisher hereby disclaims any responsibility for them.

ISBN: 978-0-595-47367-0 (pbk)
ISBN: 978-0-595-91645-0 (ebk)

Printed in the United States of America

This book is dedicated in memoriam to our loving father and husband, General Robert D. Russ, USAF (Ret) and to anyone who has ever helped further the development and advancement of people with Down Syndrome. This book would not be possible without the long hours of recollection and memories from Robin, Robert (Opey), Randy (Gooma), and Jean Russ. It is the Russ Family's hope that this book will comfort, enlighten and inspire families who have children with Down Syndrome. A special child brings a very special love.

Contents

PROLOGUE:
It's All About Love

We call him "Gooma Ya-Ya" yet no one in our family knows what it means. We know *why* we started calling our beloved brother Randy by this strange nickname, but only he knows what it means. It's a fun sounding nickname. It's hard to say without smiling, which is perfect because it's hard to be around Randy without smiling.

Born Randall Hayes Russ on April 29, 1959 to Bob and Jean Russ, he is the eldest of three children followed by Sister Robin then me, Brother Bobby. Growing up, our home was filled with love and compassion, much of which can be attributed to Gooma's insatiable desire for hugs.

There were, though, many challenges along the way. The circumstances surrounding Gooma's birth were hectic. Furthermore, efforts to educate him were often met with obstacles not solely from his disability, Down Syndrome, but more often from the ignorance and prejudices of others. But challenges hold within them rewards for those with the courage to accept and the determination and will to overcome them. On a spring night in 1997, Gooma accepted a challenge and that challenge was the inspiration for this book.

It happened at a Restaurant/Sports bar in Ft. Walton Beach, Florida. Gooma and I had just finished dinner and walked into the bar to play a couple of games of pool. The bar was very crowded. The Braves were playing the Mets and judging by the lack of high fives, the Mets were winning. A long row of quarters lined the top of both pool tables so we decided to get a soda at the bar and wait.

Just then a friend of ours, Darryl, walked up and gave Gooma a hug. He was up next on the pool table and asked us if we wanted to play, so we did. Halfway through the game, Darryl walked up to the bar to get a beer. While Darryl was at the bar, he got into an argument with a guy named Jeff. The argument got more and more heated and before long, Darryl and Jeff were standing chin to chin

1

ready to go to blows. When Gooma saw this, he put down his pool cue and walked over to Darryl and Jeff. Gooma can't stand discourse of any kind, but especially not amongst his friends.

"Hey, what's going on here?" Gooma asked.

"Go back to the pool game Gooma" Darryl quipped, "I'll be there in a minute."

Darryl then turned his attention back to Jeff. It seemed like fists were getting ready to fly, but Gooma didn't go away.

"Come on Darryl, it's your turn," Gooma said.

"Gooma! I'll be there in a minute, now please leave us alone!" Darryl said restraining his temper.

"Fighting's not the answer you know," Gooma said.

Jeff was taken back by Darryl and Gooma's conversation in the middle of what was sure to be a bar room brawl. Darryl tried to get Gooma to go away one more time, but it didn't work.

Gooma stepped in between Darryl and Jeff and wrapped his arms around Darryl, holding Darryl's arms to his side. Gooma is a very strong man. He swims 60 laps a day and his shoulders show it. When he hugs you, you can't break the hug no matter how hard you try.

"It's all about love, Darryl," Gooma said.

Darryl was annoyed and he squirmed to try to break Gooma's grip. Gooma wouldn't budge. He kept saying "It's all about love," "It's all about love." Darryl eventually stopped squirming and wrapped his arms around Gooma and gave him a hug. When Gooma finally released his grip, Darryl was calm and Jeff had gone back to his bar stool. Darryl came back to finish the game of pool.

Ten minutes later, Darryl was back at the bar sitting next to Jeff. They were toasting each other and patting each other on the back. Gooma had used the power of love to diffuse a potentially violent situation. To this day, Darryl and Jeff are good friends.

As I sat with my Mom later that night recounting the whole story in amazement, it brought up other memorable stories of life with Gooma; stories of triumph, stories of sorrow, stories of learning, stories of love. We talked for hours about the many ways Gooma has influenced the lives of our family and friends. We laughed until our stomachs hurt at some of the things he has said and done and we wept at the sorrows we've endured. We wondered aloud what life might have been like if she and Dad had heeded the "experts" advice when he was born. Life without our Gooma?

Over the next few months, with the recollections of my sister Robin, even more stories came to light. Stories we all agreed should one day be in a book.

1

The Lottery

In the Virginia suburbs of Washington, DC sits a modest two-story confederate grey home. The lawn looks like it's been to a military barber; a short, tight crew cut stands at attention and a razor sharp edge meets the sidewalk. A stepping stone path leading to the front porch winds through a rock garden where once there was a mess of overgrown ivy. There isn't a blade of grass out of line or a pebble misplaced.

Inside, at a large round pine kitchen table sit two sweaty men, one reading a newspaper, the other anxiously sifting through unopened mail. Dad and Gooma have been working in the yard all morning and now it's lunch time.

In the country style kitchen, Mom is diligently preparing sandwiches and rationing potato chips because they are loaded with fat and salt. Her high pronounced cheekbones and strong chin are somewhat tamed by her soft green eyes. She wears her grayless curly hair high like a crown and tight about her neck and ears. Around her neck hangs a pair of bifocals, which she frequently can't find.

In a sudden outburst Gooma shouts, "I can't believe it, I won! I can't believe it, I WON!"

"What's the fuss Bud?" Dad asks.

Gooma hands him the Publisher's Clearinghouse Letter and points out the bold type that clearly says, "Randy Russ, You Have Won $10 Million Dollars." Dad grins in wonderment at his son's vivid imagination before pointing out what Gooma has obviously overlooked; the small print in the bottom left corner that says, "If you have the matching code numbers."

"What's all the commotion?" says Mom as she places their sandwiches in front of them.

Gooma and Dad are noticeably disappointed that they can actually count the number of potato chips on the plate but hey, at least they got *some*.

Gooma snatches the envelope from Dad and eagerly hands it to Mom and says, "Look what it says HERE Mom." He points to the bold preferable statement and deliberately neglects the sinking disclaimer as if his fate would be changed if Mom didn't notice.

"Let's look at this after lunch," she says with a wry smile and a wink not wanting to be the deflator of dreams.

As she sits down with them and eats her half sandwich, no chips, she looks lovingly at the man-child sitting next to her. She thinks briefly about that fateful day some 35 years ago when her husband had said, "Jeanie, when you are done, please come here, I want to talk to you." In a moment she thinks of all that has and has not come to pass since. Of how the "experts" predictions went lost and how the hidden blessings came home.

After lunch, Dad heads outside to barber the back yard and says, "Come on Gooma, we're not done, we got more work to do."

Ugh! The choice between yard work with Dad or dreaming of winning $10 million dollars with Mom wasn't a difficult choice by any means. Unfortunately, it wasn't his choice.

"Alright, alright I'm coming," Randy groans as he shuffles towards the door at a speed that would cause impatience in a sloth.

Always aware and compassionate, Mom says sternly, "Now Bob, he'll be there when we're done." Rarely did she trump Dad, except when it came to Gooma.

She and Gooma spent the next five minutes looking for her glasses and the following half hour filling out the forms and weeding through the list of all the magazines one didn't have to subscribe to in order to be eligible to win. Of course anyone who has ever responded to this particular sweepstakes knows that the see through window in the postage paid return envelope clearly shows whether they are subscribing to a magazine or not. There is bound to be an assembly line somewhere where workers systematically throw out the non-subscriber's entries without even opening them.

Gooma's list of favorite magazines is quite short. It consists of only one magazine. So the sticker was affixed next to that one magazine; the one Dad had ingeniously used to help Randy practice and develop his reading and writing skills, TV Guide.

As the two of them walked ceremoniously to the mailbox to raise that little red flag, Randy was confident he was going to win. Mom was considerably less confident but there was still that nagging lingering chance. Just maybe she thought. On their way back to the house, Mom wondered aloud.

"Gooma, what would you do with 10 Million dollars?" She asked.

He stopped and thought for a moment then said, "Save it."

This tickled her and she responded with, "Oh Gooma, we won the lottery when we got you."

"What?" he said, "You won the lottery and got me?" They started walking again and he shook his head somberly and said, "You should have took the money."

2

A Sign of Things to Come

In 1959, the F-101 Voodoo was the newest and most technologically advanced fighter jet aircraft in the world. There was only one operational squadron and only the best of the best pilots got to fly it.

All of his life my Dad had been presented with challenges. He was born Robert Dale Russ, on March 7, 1933, at the height of the Great Depression. Eight short years later, he would have to help support his family after his father died. When his family moved away from Wapato, Washington his senior year in high school, he stayed above a friend's barn and worked in the apple orchard to pay his rent so he could finish at the school where he was captain of the football team. He spent his summers in Alaska working as a fisherman to pay his tuition at Washington State University where he played football, was an outstanding ROTC cadet, and was President of his Fraternity. During the school year, he worked in a local diner. All this hard work and determination wasn't enough to keep him from falling short on tuition by $1000 dollars before his senior year. So he went to a bank to borrow the money. When asked for collateral, he said all he had was his good name. The Banker replied "I am going to take a chance on you." Years later, long after Dad had paid back the loan, he found out that the banker put up the collateral to back the loan.

After graduation, he went in to the US Air Force flight-training program where he finished in the top one percent of his class. He received the coveted "Top Gun" award. Only the top one percent of flight candidates got to fly fighter planes; the rest had to settle for big bombers or air transports.

Now here he was, 1st Lieutenant Bob Russ, one of the best fighter pilots in the world, flying the best fighter plane in the world. His dedication, hard work and staunch adherence to his own personal integrity had been a good formula for success for him.

On a cold spring night in a hot F-101 somewhere over Germany, Dad got the news.

"Russ, your wife is going to have a baby. Bug out," he heard his squadron commander say over the radio.

He couldn't believe how bad the timing was. He couldn't believe the fear that had just taken hold of this fearless man. He couldn't believe he was about to break the cardinal rule of air combat by leaving his wingman, regardless of the fact that he was being given permission to do so.

"I'm out," he squawked over the radio as he banked sharply and turned the nose of his F-101 to a heading of two-eight-niner.

The flight from the training area over Germany to Bentwaters, England, was about 300 miles. Despite the fact that he was flying a jet that travels faster than the speed of sound, it seemed to him like he was stuck in rush hour traffic. It was, up until then, the longest 18 minutes of his life, yet he knew it was just the beginning of an even longer journey.

Was she in pain? Could she hold on? He remembered what she had said to him that morning as he prepared to go to work. The words that had made him alter his morning routine by gassing up their 1957 VW Beetle *before* work rather than *after*—words that he hardly believed at the time.

"Today we are going to have a baby," Mom said. He regretted how callous his response had been.

The landing was perfect as usual. Even in the midst of anxiety and excitement, he was the consummate professional. As he drove off the base, he noticed the reminder sign posted at the gate. "Readiness is our Profession"; He was glad he had gassed up the VW on the way in.

Ten minutes later, he arrived at their one bedroom base house that came pre-furnished by the military in the avocado green and pumpkin orange décor of the era. Their living room was a conversation pit style with a hard couch and a couple of easy chairs adorning a kidney shaped coffee table with ashtrays on each end. A small black and white TV with an almost circular screen that didn't get much use sat in the corner.

She was sitting in *his* chair. She looked up and with a grin, said, "I told you today was the day."

"Fine, now go make my breakfast," was his reply that morning when she said *'Today we are going to have a baby'*. Dad said he was only kidding, but she had heard it enough before to know he was at least half serious.

◆   ◆   ◆

On a typical day, they woke up early around 5am. Mom fixed a hot breakfast as most dutiful housewives did in the years before bra burning and the ERA. Dad read the paper, and then headed off to defend the free world. Mom cleaned house, did the laundry, and leafed through the Betty Crocker cookbook. She attended the many "not required, but highly recommended" wives' club meetings and luncheons and occasionally played bridge with the neighborhood gals. There were no shops or shopping centers. They were out in the country.

Dad had to go TDY (Temporary Duty) to Africa three times a year, six weeks at a time, for bombing and gunnery practice. Mom was very lonely during these times and resented the isolation. Before they were married she had been a Stewardess—not a flight attendant—she'll tell you, for United Airlines. She traveled extensively and loved the excitement, but now she was stuck in the tiny town of Aldeburg in the southeast corner of Suffolk England on the North Sea. To make matters worse, her parents lived 5,000 miles away in San Francisco.

When Dad wasn't TDY, he would be home around 5:30 PM, eager for dinner and the evening paper. He would find *his* easy chair and wait to see what Betty Crocker had inspired Mom to prepare. He was sure it wouldn't be salmon loaf. He had instructed her never to put that on the table again. After dinner, Mom would do the dishes while Dad prepared for the next day's work. Then it was off to bed, so they could wake up and do the same things tomorrow.

◆   ◆   ◆

"Are you ok?" he asked as he helped his pregnant wife out of *his* chair. "How far apart are the contractions?"

"They're still far enough apart that I think we can make it," she said, "but we better get going."

Dad helped Mom into the front seat of the VW, and then went back into the house to gather the bags that he had packed earlier that morning, just in case. *Readiness is our Profession.*

The nearest hospital with a maternity ward was eight hours away in the town of Wimpole Park in Cambridgeshire. Their doctor at the Aldeburg Clinic had made them do a dry run six weeks earlier just to make sure they wouldn't get lost when the big day came. He gave them a map of the English countryside; complete with marked waypoints where midwives were located, just in case.

Off they went, twisting and turning their way through the English countryside, over rolling green hills, and through tiny towns that had been there for centuries. The roads were mostly dirt and the ones that were paved, were paved with stones. That old VW danced on those roads like a drop of water on a hot griddle. Every protruding rock had its alter ego pothole. Dad silently wished his F-101 was a two-seater.

He figured that from the time he got the call on the radio from his squadron commander earlier that morning over Germany, to the time they would reach the hospital he would have traveled almost 600 miles. The first leg of the trip took 18 minutes; the last leg would take eight hours.

When they finally reached the hospital, Dad was exhausted and Mom was ready. He paced nervously outside the delivery room like most men who are about to be fathers for the first time. But there was one additional worry. He was worried about something else. Several months earlier Dad's sister Carol had a baby. She told him that the woman in the adjoining room had a *Mongoloid* baby. Mongoloid or Mongolism was the medical term used before the condition was renamed Down Syndrome. At the time, he had no idea what a mongoloid baby was and he didn't want to know. All he knew was that it sounded bad.

When the Doctor emerged from the delivery room with Randy, he said, "Congratulations Lt. Russ, you have a son!"

"He's not a mongoloid baby is he?" Dad asked.

The doctor later admitted that he wondered if Dad had noticed something he hadn't, so he carried Randy into the nursery and took a closer look. Sure enough, he saw a few symptoms that were normally associated with Mongolism, yet he was not sure. Further testing was needed but he didn't want to alarm the new dad.

In the late fifties, there wasn't a blood test for Down Syndrome. Observation of physical characteristics was used to diagnose the condition. Without a blood test, the only way to be sure was to wait until the child was further developed and examine him again.

So Dad, Mom and Randy packed into their VW and headed for home. Like most new parents, they delighted in showing off their pride and joy. They took countless pictures and strolls through their neighborhood. They invited all of their friends to the house to see their new wonder.

Many of the friends they met in England are still friends today—Sammy and Chet Lamb, Bob and Dell Stone. The Stones are Randy's God Parents and the two couples have supported our family with their love and friendship from the very beginning to the present day.

Six weeks later, the doctor called to schedule a check-up. They would have to take that long ride once again. It never crossed their minds that a local doctor could do the compulsory check up. The truth was that the doctor wanted to test for Mongolism.

The doctor told Dad first. Very little research had been done on the subject and what little had been done suggested a grim outlook. Dad was told his son might not walk or talk, much less read and write. He might not learn to feed himself or even go to the bathroom by himself. The worst news of all was that his life span probably wouldn't be very long. The doctor told Dad that according to all the "experts" it was in their best interest to institutionalize Randy and forget him. Dad and Mom were young and could have more babies.

The next question was who would tell Mom. Dad decided it would be best if the news came from him. He wasn't sure how or when he would tell her. He needed some time to think. The trip back to Aldeburg seemed agonizingly long for Dad. The whole way home Mom held Randy and chatted gleefully unaware of his condition, while Dad drove quiet and pensive.

That night Dad was "pulling alert." Pulling alert was a term used by fighter pilots. Similar to "standing guard," it meant he would sit in his F-101 alone at the end of a runway and wait for orders to take off. So Dad sat there at the end of that runway, prepared to take off at a moments notice and fight whatever evil threatened the free world. The order never came. He sat there only with the company of his confounded thoughts, and he wept.

How would he handle *this* challenge?

Dad was a man who achieved success by following the manual. He was a "manual guy," through and through. One of Dad's biggest pet peeves was when someone tried to assemble something without reading the instructions. Dad believed if you followed the instructions and worked hard, you could accomplish anything.

With Randy, there was no formula for success and no manual to follow. No amount of planning, hard work and perseverance would change the fact that his son was a *Mongoloid*. For the first time in his life, there was a problem that didn't have a predefined solution.

The next evening, Dad sat in the den reading the paper as Mom did the dishes.

"Jeannie, when you're done in there, please come here. I need to talk to you," he said.

It sounded a little ominous. She wondered if he was going to scold her for something. She quickly finished the dishes and went to his side.

"The doctor said there's something wrong with Randy," he said.

Her heart hit a brick wall. In a split second, her life changed forever. Every malady, from polio to leprosy flashed through her mind; every malady except one. It was the longest second of her life.

"He has symptoms consistent with mongolism," Dad said.

What on earth was mongolism? She was soon to become an expert. Dad explained what the doctor had told him. When all was said and done, she went to Randy. She held him with a type of restrictive tenderness that only a mother can.

The tears began to flow. What would this life have in store for them? Mom and Dad struggled with the grim outlook. They didn't know what they were going to do, but they knew what they were NOT going to do. They weren't going to institutionalize their baby.

If the "experts" said Randy would never learn to talk, they would do everything in their power to make sure Randy would speak his mind. If the "experts" said Randy would never read, they were going to do everything in their power to teach their son to read. One of Dad's favorite sayings was, "The only way to be certain you can't achieve is to not try."

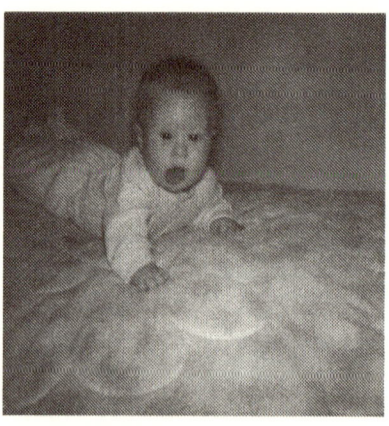

As Mom held Randy, she said to him "You are going to be the best that you can be!" and she vowed it with every fiber of her being.

The tears in her eyes evaporated from the heat of her determination. Mom, once happy in her acquiescence, would eventually become a leader. Their lives, and the lives of many others, changed in that one moment.

Randy Age 6 Months

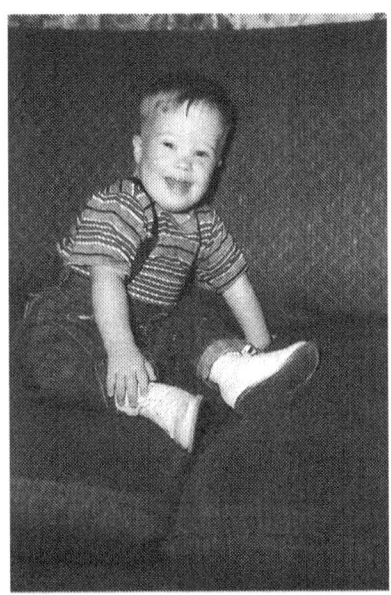

Randy Age 2

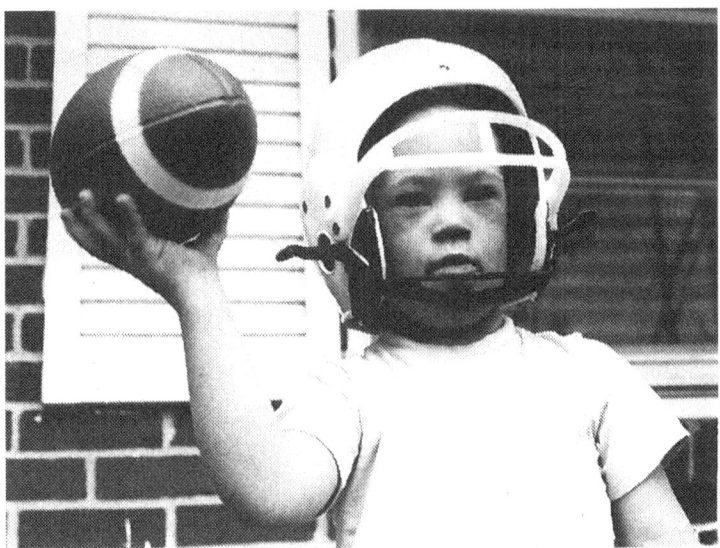

Range Age 6

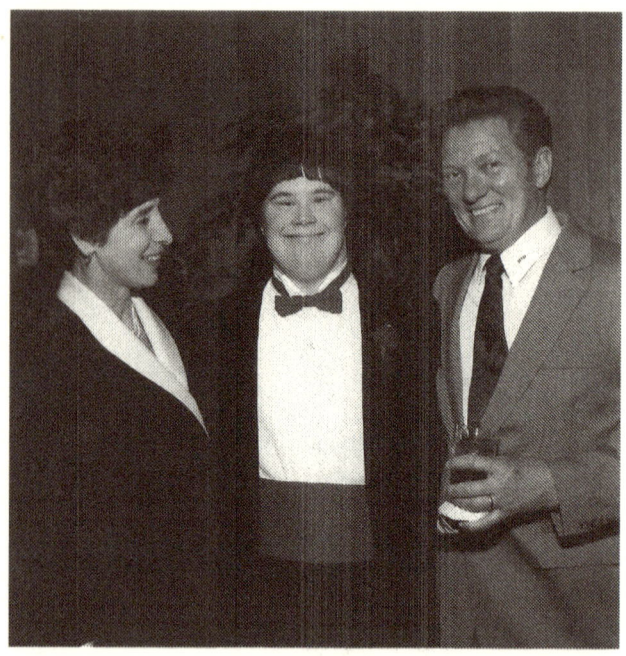

Randy's God Parents—Dell and Robert Stone (Randy Age 25)

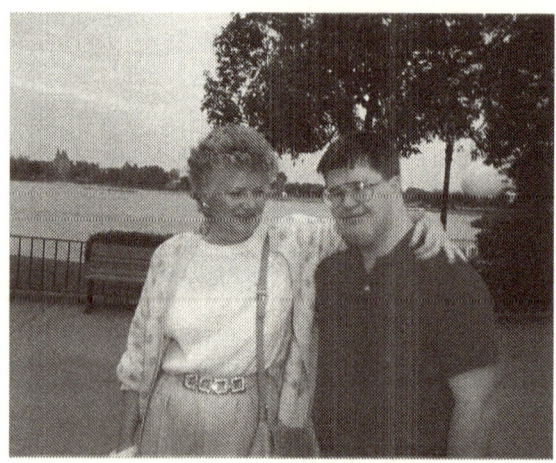

Randy & Sammy (Randy Age 33)

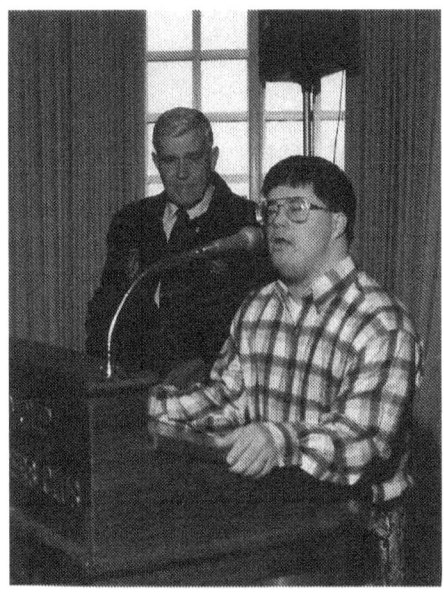

Randy gives a speech at Air Force luncheon

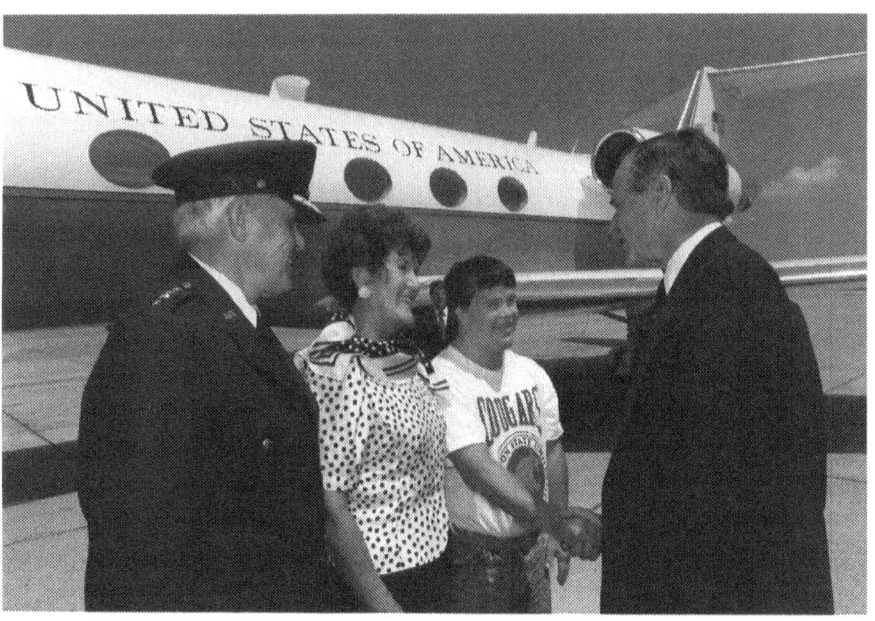

Randy and President Bush

3

The History and Science of Down Syndrome

(There are many books and resources on the Internet that explain the technical, medical, and scientific aspects of Down Syndrome. Here is a brief overview of the condition and its history. For more detailed information and links to more resources, please go to *www.ndsccenter.org*.)

Down Syndrome is named for a 19th century English physician, Dr. John Langdon Haydon Down, M.D. who worked with children with learning disabilities and unusual physical markers in the 1860s. In his paper titled, "Observations on an Ethnic Classification of Idiots"[1], Dr. Down used the terms Mongolism and Mongolian Idiocy to describe these children partly because of their somewhat Asian-appearing eyes. By the 20th century, "Mongolian Idiocy" had become the most recognizable form of mental retardation. Most people with it were institutionalized. Few of the associated medical problems were treated, and most died in infancy or early adult life.[2] Some states instituted programs of involuntary sterilization. Even more extreme, was the Nazi euthanasia program called "Aktion T-4" where between 75,000 to 250,000 people with Down Syndrome and other mental and physical disabilities were systematically slaughtered to promote "racial hygiene."

People with Down Syndrome would be referred to as Mongoloids until 1961 when a group of geneticists suggested the term be renamed Down's Syndrome. In 1965, the World Health Organization dropped Mongolism as a reference to the disorder at the request of the Mongolian delegate. In 1975, the United States

---

1. Down, J.L.H. (1866). "Observations on an ethnic classification of idiots." Clinical Lecture Reports, London Hospital 3: 259-262.
2. Wikipedia, http://en.wikipedia.org/wiki/History_of_Down_syndrome

National Institute of Health recommended eliminating the possessive form of the name since Dr. Down neither had nor owned the disorder; however, Down's Syndrome is still used in England and some other countries.

Little was known about the origins of Down Syndrome until 1959, the year Randy was born, when Professor Jérôme Lejeune discovered that the condition resulted from an extra 21st chromosome. In a typically developed person, there are 23 pairs of chromosomes. During the formation of the egg or the sperm, each pair of chromosomes splits so that only one chromosome is contained in each egg or sperm. With Down Syndrome, the 21st chromosome pair does not split and a double dose of chromosomes goes to the affected egg or sperm.

Medically, science does not know what triggers that extra 21st chromosome. It is known that the chromosome in question produces some extra proteins, which cause some of the typical physical features of persons with Down Syndrome. Science still does not know which proteins are involved, or how they actually cause Down Syndrome.

Some of the physical characteristics include folds over the eyes, a flattened bridge of the nose, a single palmal crease, and decreased muscle tone. They also generally have small mouths and enlarged tongues, making for challenging speech issues. In addition, many people with Down Syndrome have congenital heart defects which in the past, if left untreated, contributed to their relatively short life spans. Today, with early intervention and proper medical treatment—and if they have lots of love, good nutrition, exercise, and positive social interaction—they have a good chance of living a long, productive life.

There are several types of Down Syndrome. *Trisomy 21*, the most common, occurs in about 95% of cases and happens when every cell in the body has an extra 21st chromosome. *Mosaicism*, like Gooma, is rare with only 1-2% occurrence and is where some cells in the body have an extra 21st chromosome, but others do not. Gooma has some, but not all, of the typical physical characteristics. For instance, he has normal palmal creases, better developed nervous and circulatory systems, and no heart defects. The other two types are *Robertsonian translation*, often referred to as familial Down Syndrome, which is rare but has a high degree of heredity; and *Duplication of a Portion of Chromosome 21*, which is extremely rare and happens when only a portion of the 21st chromosome splits in the egg or sperm.

In the United States, about one baby in a thousand is born with Down Syndrome. There are no associations between Down Syndrome and any given culture, ethnic group, socioeconomic status, or geographic region. The odds of having a baby with Down Syndrome for a mother less than 25 years of age is about one in 1,400. By age 35, the odds rise to one in 350. By age 40, the odds rise again to one in 100. The chances of a parent with one Down Syndrome child having a second child with Down's are approximately one in 100.

Before the discovery of the chromosomal causes of Down Syndrome it was believed that it was caused by trauma during pregnancy. Today, aside from the association between the age of the mother and the likelihood of having a baby with Down Syndrome, no other causes or correlations have been identified or proven.

In the past, parents only knew they had a child with Down Syndrome after birth. Today, there are several types of prenatal tests available. The most common are amniocentesis and chorionic villus sampling (CVS). In amniocentesis, a needle is inserted into the belly of the mother into the womb, to sample fetal cells in the amniotic fluid. This fluid is then sent for chromosome analysis. This test is usually performed between the 14th and 18th weeks of pregnancy and carries with it a risk of miscarriage. The CVS process, on the other hand, involves sampling cells from the chorionic villi, a structure in the womb that has fetal cells, but is not the fetus itself. This test is done between 9 and 12 weeks, and is often done in conjunction with the amniocentesis. The CVS test is estimated to detect approximately 35% of fetuses with Down Syndrome after confirmation by amniocentesis.

4

The Education of Gooma

The morning after Dad told Mom about Gooma's condition, she woke up with the feeling there was something wrong. As she became more awake, reality hit her and she thought, *my baby is* a *Mongoloid.* The coming months would be very difficult. She was comforted only by the strength of her resolve and Dad at her side.

Mom knew nothing about Mongolism, so she started to do research. The first book she read was by Roy Rodgers and Dale Evens titled, "Angel Unaware." The famous movie stars had had a mongoloid child. She admits that in a strange way, it was comforting to know that this could happen to famous people like them. Sadly, Roy and Dale's child passed away before she was two years old. This fact only deepened Mom's fears.

She had virtually no support system. She didn't know anyone who had a special needs child and the one person, other than Dad; she knew she could lean on, her mother, lived 5,000 miles away in San Francisco. So she searched for support.

She wrote to the Association for Retarded Citizens in New York and they mailed her some pamphlets. The pamphlets weren't much help. She went to many small English churches in search of anyone with whom she could relate. Finally she found a church with a small group of parents who had children with Down Syndrome. One of the children was in his teens, happy, and in good health. This gave Mom hope. She enjoyed the company of this group, until something happened that would be a recurring theme in her life. Dad got orders and they would have to move.

The orders would take them to Oxnard, California. Though she would miss her support group, Mom was excited about moving closer to her parents. San Francisco was only a few hours drive from Oxnard and she couldn't wait for her mother to meet her baby boy. Unfortunately, that would never happen. Her mother passed away before they arrived in Oxnard. Her father did get to see Randy, but only once. He passed away a year later.

Her sadness would be tempered by a new joy, she was pregnant again. She and Dad worried that their new baby might have Down Syndrome. On September 28, 1960, Robin Dell Russ was born. The moment she was born, Mom asked the Doctor if the baby was "normal." His answer made her cry. In those days, expecting fathers didn't go into the delivery room. Standing right outside the door, Dad heard Mom's cries and he feared. When the doctor came out and told Dad that Robin was a beautiful baby girl and that she didn't have Down Syndrome, Dad realized that Mom was crying tears of joy, and he wept.

They wouldn't be in Oxnard very long. They moved to Hamilton, California for a short stint and then to Montgomery, Alabama where Randy would be introduced to public education and Mom would be introduced to bureaucracy.

Mom tried to get Randy into a preschool but he was a year older than the age limit, so the administrator wouldn't allow it. Randy wasn't ready for kindergarten, much less first grade, but Mom was determined to get him in. She joined forces with a teacher who was sympathetic to her plight.

In a meeting with the administrator and Mom, this teacher stood up and with reference to her students said, "I don't think five years old is too young for a lesson in tolerance."

Randy was in school and he was learning. This teacher was good with Randy and Mom noticed him making progress. It's too bad it didn't last.

In 1965, our family moved to Colorado. Mom would have to start over again. Mom called the Special Education Department and asked where he could go to school. They said he could not go anywhere until he was seven. She told them she would enroll him in the nearest grade school like any other child. They said "You can't do that" and she replied "Watch me."

She demanded they allow Randy to take a placement test and he performed very well on it. With test results in hand and much lobbying, she was able to convince a majority of the school board to let him in. As a result, Randy was the first

Down Syndrome child ever mainstreamed into the public school system in Colorado.

Things were looking up. He excelled in the new school. Mom and Dad decided they wanted one more child and on February 23 1966, I was born Robert William Russ. Two years later, Dad got orders again. Only this time the orders were different. Mom and the kids couldn't go with him. These orders sent Dad to Vietnam, to war.

Mom was alone with three children; living with the daily fear that her husband might not make it home. Most of the men in the neighborhood were in Vietnam at the time, so Mom and the other wives would get together to support each other. Dad had been gone for almost a year and a half when Mom got some dreadful news. Dad's plane had been shot down over enemy territory. In the movies, it's common to see a blue military staff car pull into the driveway to notify the family that their loved one was killed or injured. This wasn't the movies. Mom never saw a staff car. She read about it in "The Air Force Times" newspaper, days after it happened. Luckily, Dad was rescued and she received a letter from him a week later telling her all about it.

Dad had flown 240 combat missions before being shot down. He flew two more missions and then was sent home.

Dad's time away at war was tough on all of us, but especially on Randy. His teacher called Mom shortly after Dad went to war and asked if there was something wrong at home. He was just not acting like his cheery self. He was glum and grumpy and uncharacteristically somber. Mom told her where Dad was. Randy didn't understand where Dad was or why he was gone. He just knew his Daddy wasn't home. After a year, it must have seemed to Randy like Dad was never coming back.

The day that Dad came back, we met his plane as it taxied into a hanger on the Air Force Base. When Dad stepped off the plane, he looked at Randy and with outstretched arms and a quiver in his voice said, "Come here big boy!"

Randy stood motionless for a few moments gazing at his Dad with a look of joyous confusion on his face. The rest of us waited quietly, with jaws dropped for his reaction. He broke the silence saying softly and in a tone of disbelief, "Dad?"

A second later, he burst toward Dad and leapt into his arms and the sobbing began.

Dad was promoted during the war and got orders to work at the Pentagon in Washington, DC. So the family packed into our 1966 Volkswagen Bug—Mom and Dad in front, Randy and Robin in the back, and me in the cubby hole behind them—and we drove cross country.

We lived in the suburbs of Maryland outside Washington, DC. Mom got Randy enrolled without much trouble in a special education class in the public school system. One day, Mom stopped by his class to check on him and found him and the other special needs children mulling around with no structure or attention; some of them with soiled pants. The teacher was sitting at her desk reading a newspaper oblivious to what was going on. Mom complained to the principal of the school and asked for a new teacher. The principal denied her request so she and Dad went to the superintendent of schools and fought the issue. The end result was Randy got a new teacher and as usual, not long after, Dad got new orders.

Sumter, South Carolina was next. Mom was becoming a pro at navigating the bureaucracy of a public school system. However, in this town, a special education class didn't exist. The superintendent said there wasn't a demand for the class, but if she could find 20 special needs children, whose parents were willing to send them to class, then he would make it happen. Mom liked him and believed he was sincere, so she started recruiting.

Anytime she saw a handicapped child, she would explain to the parents what the superintendent had said. She found people in a variety of places from shopping malls to grocery stores to hair salons. Some of the parents were receptive to the idea, some weren't. Mom pressed on until she got firm commitments from 20 families.

Mom had been right about the superintendent. He honored his word and at the start of school in the fall of that year, a new special education class was available. However, Gooma wouldn't get to attend a single day. A month before the class started, Dad got promoted to Colonel and we moved to Goldsboro, North Carolina.

In Goldsboro, Dad was the Wing Commander of Seymour Johnson Air Force Base, the senior ranking officer. An Air Force Base is much like a city. Much of Dad's day was focused on running the military aspects of the base; the pilots, the planes and the people who support the mission. But there are also non-military aspects to a base, such as the hospital, dental clinic, church, youth clubs, and child care centers that need to be managed. With Dad's encouragement, Mom attended meetings and helped work the important issues within the societal framework of the base. Mom's responsibilities were similar to those of the First Lady, only on a smaller scale.

By chance, she met a young Lieutenant's wife who had a child with Down Syndrome. Mom remembered how difficult things had been for her almost 20 years earlier so she helped the woman. Mom soon learned that as the Commander's wife, she could help effect change on a system and not just for herself. She helped institute programs that aided base families with disabled children get the help that she didn't get when she was younger.

Over the next eight years, our family moved five more times. In 1985, Dad was promoted to Four Star General and became Commander of the Tactical Air Command (TAC) on Langley Air Force Base in Hampton, Virginia. At the time, the Air Force was structured into three main commands. TAC was all the fighter planes. SAC (Strategic Air Command) was all the bomber airplanes and MAC (Military Airlift Command) was all of the transport airplanes. What he once did for a single Air Force Base in Goldsboro, he was now responsible for doing for some 21 bases located throughout the world.

Mom continued her involvement with the non-military aspects of all of these bases. She gave particular attention to helping families with special needs children. She instituted a program that provided a Forward Outreach Worker or FOW as they called them. When a family with a special needs child arrived at any base in TAC, they were immediately assigned an FOW to help with any of the special issues these families faced.

It is quite common for the Air Force to honor a retired General by naming a building or a street after them. What's not common is for the Air Force to honor a retired General's wife in the same manner. As a testament to Mom's efforts, on November 14, 2003, the new state-of-the-art child development center on Langley Air Force Base was dedicated and named the "General Bob and Jean Russ Child Development Center."

By the time Randy reached his 20's he was able to read and write on a high school level. Mom and Dad's diligent efforts to prove the "experts" wrong were successful. Now it was time for Randy to become a productive member of society and join the work force. This would present Mom with a new set of challenges.

Initially, he worked at a sheltered workshop putting together gift baskets and such. This was fine for a while, but the work was repetitive and boring. Randy would come home dragging his feet with his head hung low. Mom knew this wasn't good for him, so she signed him up with an employment agency that specialized in finding jobs for people with disabilities. Weeks went by with no results.

Not being one to wait on fate, Mom took Randy to apply for a job bussing tables and washing dishes at a popular Mexican restaurant just outside the base. The manager turned them down, but Mom was persistent. She was confident that Randy would do a good job, so she offered to train and even pay for him to work there. He reluctantly agreed.

Over the next few days, people from the base would come in for lunch and see Randy and Mom in their aprons, bussing tables and washing dishes. On one occasion, a young military officer asked her, "Aren't you General Russ' wife?"

"Yes," she replied.

"Well, what are you doing working here," he asked.

"Times are tough," she said, and went back to work.

Randy learned quickly and she hung up her apron not long after. As agreed, she took a check to the manager to pay for Randy's employment each week. Several weeks later, the manager told her he could not accept any more of her money. She thought he was going to let Randy go, but instead, he said that Randy was one of his best workers and that he was going to put him on the payroll.

Randy loved working at that restaurant. The staff loved him and so did the customers. He was there for a couple of years before Dad got orders.

From then on, Randy worked at a number of places. Mom always went and trained him if necessary. Currently, he works at an Albertsons grocery store and a Burger King restaurant in Shalimar, Florida. He recently came home from Albertsons with a framed certificate and $50.00 for being the most courteous employee.

At Albertsons, some customers will stand in a longer line, just to have him take their groceries to their car. Often, people want to tip him but Albertsons has a no tip policy. Dad role-played with him to make sure he didn't violate this policy.

Dad said "Randy, you are the bagger and I'll be the customer. Thank you for helping me, here's a tip."

"No thank you," Randy said.

"Oh come on, I want you to have it," Dad pressed.

"Okay," Randy said.

"No. No! Randy, don't take the tip no matter what," Dad said. They would have to try again. This time Dad tried a different approach, "You have been such a big help with my groceries, and I would like to give you a tip."

"No thank you!" Randy said.

"Oh come on, I want you to have it," Dad pressed.

"Absolutely not," Randy said.

Dad took the money and put it in Randy's pocket and said "Please take it."

Randy said "Okay."

This went on several more times until Randy finally got it—No matter what they say, don't take the money.

Most anywhere he goes in town, someone will recognize him from Albertsons or Burger King and stop and chat. He has really become somewhat of a local celebrity.

When Gooma was born in 1959, there was very little support for families of people with Down Syndrome. Today, the good news is that there are many national support groups, with local branches, and on the Internet. Also, many children with Down Syndrome are in regular classrooms, and adults with Down Syndrome work and are productive members of society.

Randy's education far exceeds any expectations placed upon him at birth. He has been our teacher as well.

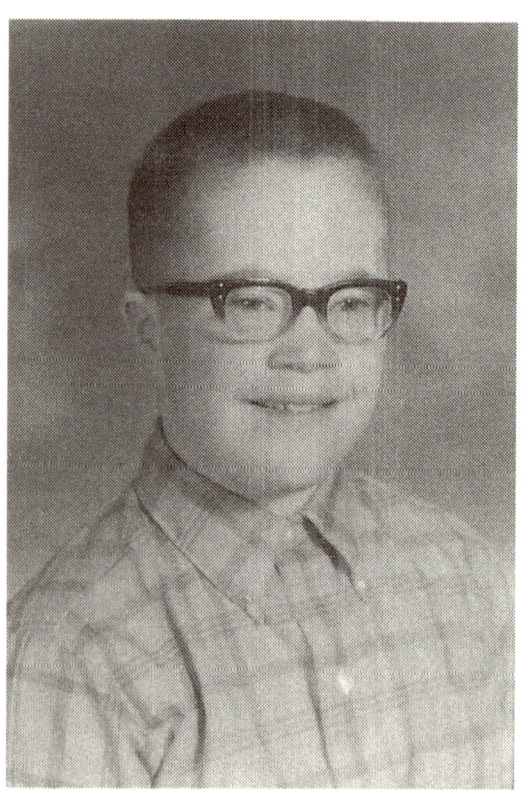

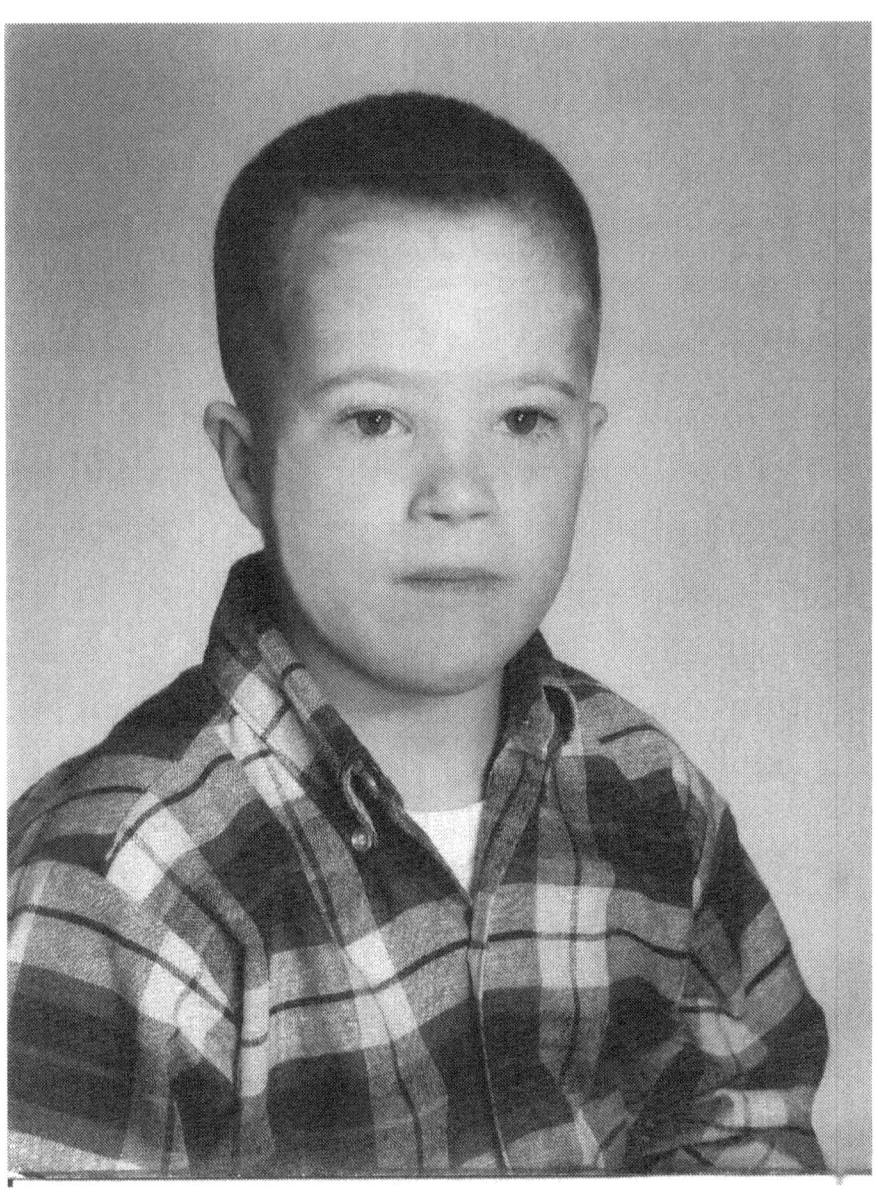

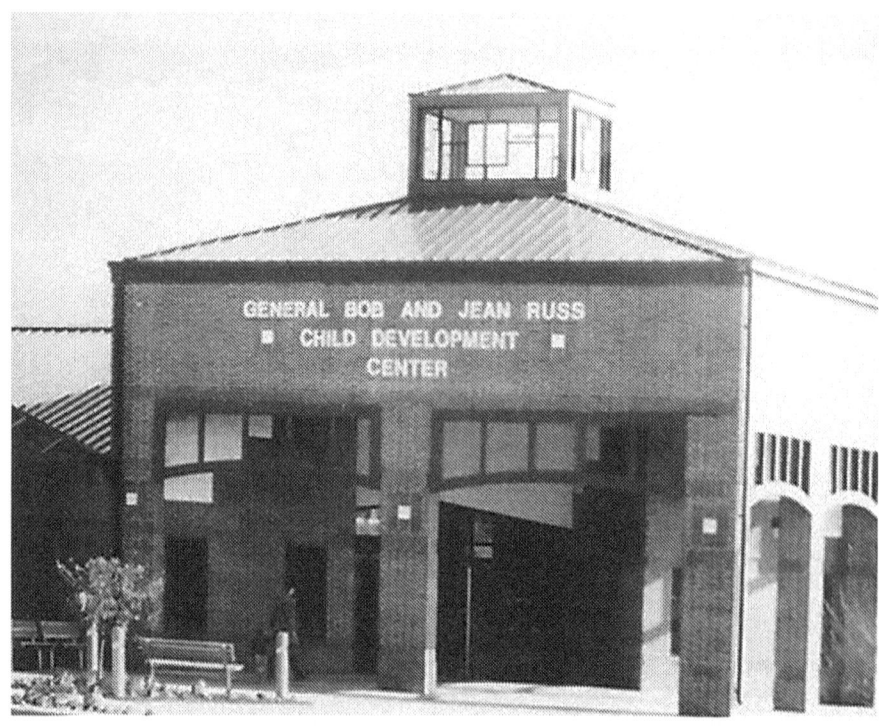

Child Development Center at Langley AFB Named after Mom and Dad

5

Recollections from Sis, by Robin Russ Lindenmeier

I was born 18 months after Randy. My Grandma told my Mom that she always loved the name Robin, and so I was named. Unfortunately, I never got to meet my Grandma. She died before I was born. As I grew older, Randy and I were like two peas-in-a-pod. For a while, we were the same developmental age as each other. However, I started to surpass Randy on the developmental scale and became his bigger sister. Five years later, my brother Bobby was born.

Mom and Dad had to give Randy a lot of extra attention because of his disability, not realizing that I was beginning to feel a little left out. I remember feeling that this was so unfair. I never demanded anything from my parents and all the attention went to Randy. I didn't understand that Randy needed more attention because he was special. And then to make matters worse, Bobby came along, a new baby.

I was closer to Randy than anyone realized. I'd lay awake at night trying to think of ideas to gain my parents attention. Then one night, the light bulb lit up. One of Mom and Dad's main frustrations with Randy was his speech. In the early years, it was very difficult to understand him. Mom and Dad would often remark "What is he saying?" or "What does he need?" I figured I would be his interpreter and Mom and Dad would pay more attention to me.

One day, Randy reached for the refrigerator and said "BaBaGyGu." Mom and Dad were obviously perplexed so I nonchalantly said, "He wants a popsicle."

"You can understand him?" they asked.

"Sure," I replied. So Randy got a popsicle and *so did I.*

On another day, Gooma was watching TV and said "Gagafyginggo." Mom and Dad both turned to me and said "Robin, what is he saying?"

"He wants to watch 'Casper the Friendly Ghost'," I said. It was my favorite cartoon.

From then on anytime he said something they would look to me for the answer. This was great until Mom got him a speech therapist and he learned to speak more clearly. Then I had to start devising another plan.

Randy Gets a Nickname

A lot of Randy's expression of love and happiness came through his music. He loves to sing and his favorite group is the Partridge Family. He would play their records and sit on the floor and beat on two bibles with wooden spoons as if he were playing the drums. He didn't understand the words so he created his own chorus to each of the songs he listened too. He would bang on those two bibles over and over again singing "Gooma Gooma Ya Ya."

This was a lot like listening to a dog howl at the moon, but we tolerated it because we knew he loved to sing. I told Mom and Dad that I believed the words Gooma Gooma Ya Ya meant "I love to sing" and the "Ya Ya" at the end of each Gooma, was his musical instruments playing. Mom and Dad figured I must know what he means, so Randy's nickname was formed—Gooma Ya Ya. Later it was shortened to Gooma and later on it was shortened even more too just Goom or even Goom Bag. My nickname was Bean Bag. I received my nickname from a Costa Rican Exchange Student that came to live with us. She could not pronounce Robin so she would say "Robeen." My nickname started as Bean, then Beana, and finally evolved to Bean Bag.

When I was ten, I wanted to see if there was any meaning to the word Gooma and looked up the word in the encyclopedia. There is a word Gooma. I was hoping it would mean love, hope, and friendship but it means "Australian shrub." It's also the name of a small town outside of Toyko.

Randy Goes to Junior High

Dad received orders to move to North Carolina when Randy and I were just starting Junior High School. This was a tough time for Randy and me. We went to school at Greenwood Junior High and would walk to and from school together. Some of the kids were very cruel. They used to walk behind us and call us the "Retard Twins" and throw rocks at our feet. I remember thinking, how could anyone be so cruel. I grew up with Randy and in my book; he was just like everyone else, even better.

One day, Randy was walking beside me and his shoulders dropped and his head hung low. I asked him what was wrong. Just then the usual bullies walked up behind us and stepped on our shoe heels so that our feet would come out. Randy said "That's what's wrong." I turned around and told the kids that if they did not stop there would be a big problem with their parents and the school. Just then a car pulled up with one of the kid's parents asking if there was a problem. The kids said "No problem Mom"; we were just passing Robin and Randy. I did not say anything. This time, because the situation ended. I turned to Randy and said, "I always want you to hold your head high because you are a wonderful person and we are better than they are. Don't let them get you down, they are not nice kids." I was Randy's defender in and out of school but I wasn't a very good fighter. Some times I would deck a kid for making fun of Randy and I would end up on the wrong end of the stick.

One time I came home with a black eye and told Mom that I had run into a door at school by accident. Another day I went to meet Randy after school but he wasn't at our designated meeting place. I waited for about five minutes and then went looking for him. I was frantic, where could he be? He knew that I was to meet him at this place every day. I started envisioning the worst, until I spotted him surrounded by a bunch of kids by the gym. They were telling him to pull his pants down. They said if he did, he would have a lot of friends. I caught him with his pants half-way down to his knees. Once again the great defender protected and ended up with some bruises.

My biggest concern was Randy and his self-esteem. There was no way that I was going to let bullies take charge of our lives and injure Randy's concept of self-worth. I wanted to tell Mom and Dad, but I knew they would go to the principal and the bullies would know I turned them in. I was really worried about the potential repercussions.

I finally made up my mind that I would tell. One night after dinner, I said to Dad and Mom, "there is something I have to tell you about Randy and me."

Dad said that first he had some news to tell us. He got orders and we were moving to Virginia. At that moment, my worries went away and there was a sudden feeling of relief and excitement.

"Now, What is it that you wanted to tell us?" Dad said.

"Nothing really, I just wanted to tell you about our day." I replied.

The Virginia kids were a lot nicer to us so we put the bullies behind us and move forward.

My Relationship with Randy and Food

Randy loves to eat. His whole day revolves around food. The first thing he wants to know when he wakes up is what's for breakfast. While eating breakfast, he talks about what's for lunch. During lunch, he talks about, "What are we going to have for lunch?" At lunch, he talks about "What are we going to have for dinner?" At dinner, he talks about "What are we going to have for breakfast?" People with Down Syndrome have the propensity to be overweight unless there is some intervention. Given the opportunity, Randy would eat non stop. On Sundays, Mom records his weight and they talk about. For the most part, his weight will fluctuate up or down no more than a pound or two. One Sunday, he weighed in and had gained two pounds.

"Randy, how did you gain so much?", Mom asked.

"I only eat what you fix me," he replied.

He was right! Mom tries to fix him healthy meals and make sure he doesn't overindulge but when they go out to eat he usually orders French fries.

Mom called me to ask my advice on the situation. She didn't want to deny him one of his favorite foods forever so I recommended she apply moderation and tell Randy he could have french fries only one day a week. The next day she asked him to pick the one day a week when he could have french fries. He thought about it for a minute then said with a grin—"Monday's." Mom chuckled, she realized it was Monday.

Every Sunday, Randy calls me with the "Weight Report" and says guess what tomorrow is? I reply, "happy french fry day." He replies, "You betcha."

Lessons from Randy and Mom

I learned much from being Randy's sister. I took care of him a lot, so I learned to be responsible at an early age. Thanks to Randy, I consider myself a giving, caring, loving person with an extra measure of compassion for people. I didn't realize it at the time, but my Mom's efforts to educate Randy would be an inspiration to me when I had my own children.

My husband Clark and I have a son Ryan, who had a difficult birth, which caused some developmental problems. With the perseverance and determination I learned from Mom and Dad and the support of my husband, I faced these problems with confidence and conviction. Clark and I challenged diagnoses, rejected the negative, and vowed to do whatever it took to help him. For that reason, I got a Masters Degree in Education.

Ryan graduated from high school and is now in his first year of college at the local community college. He has a Black Belt in Tae Kwon Do. His sister Sarah is equally impressive and they are generous and helpful with anyone in need, including animals. Randy has impacted the whole clan.

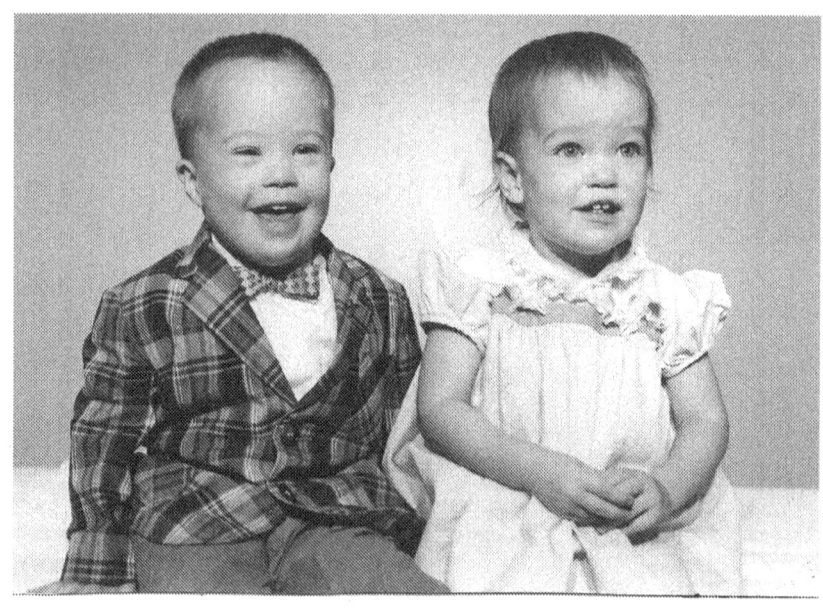

Randy and Robin

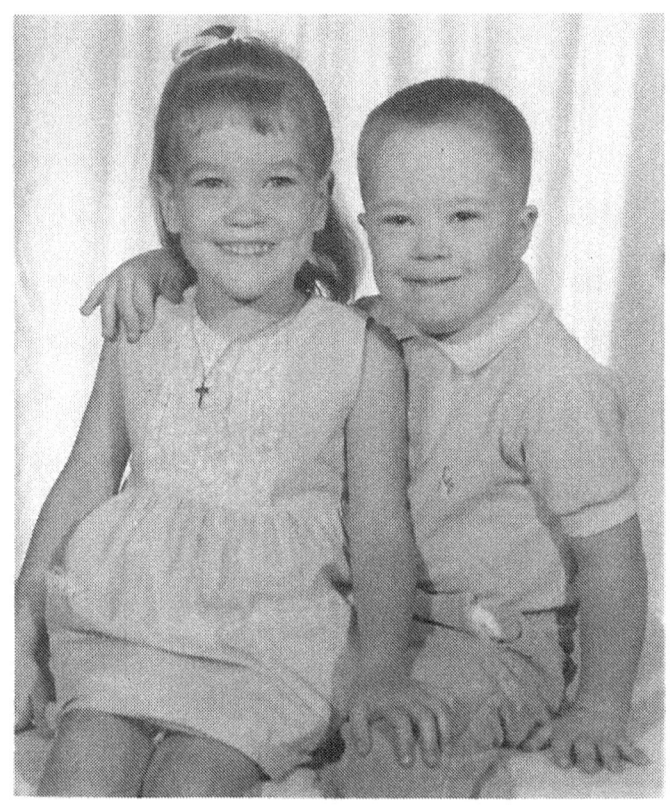

Randy and Robin

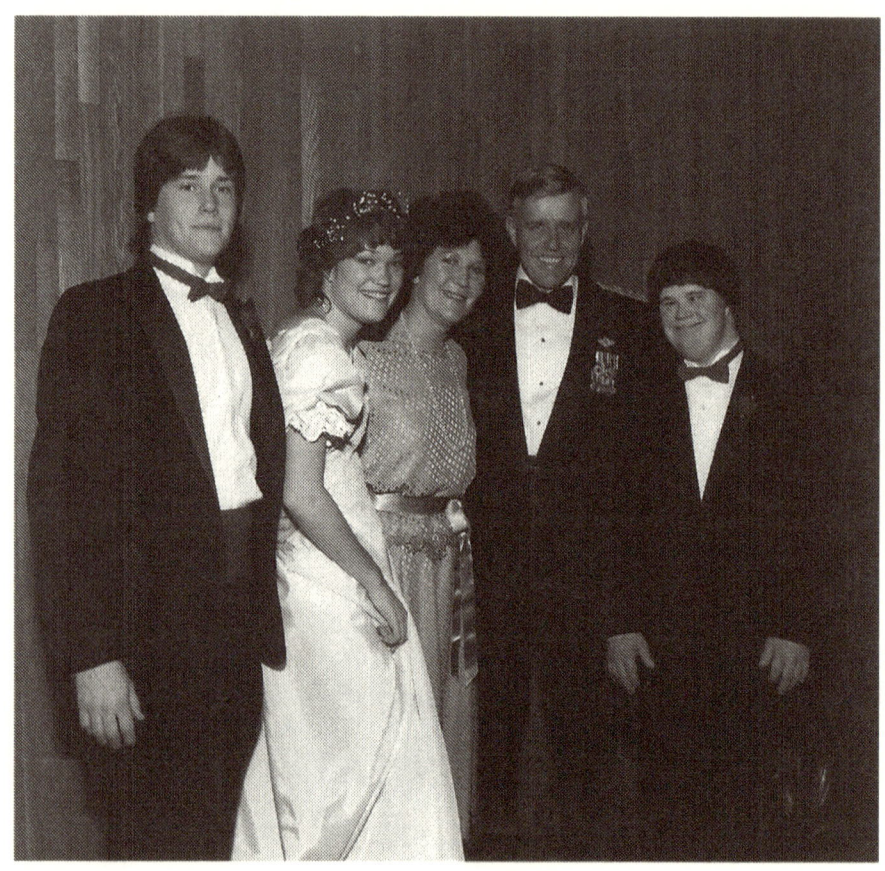

Robin's Wedding (Feb 04)

6

Three Brothers in One

Have you ever dreamed of being a kid again? What would it be like if you could just cast away the cares of your adulthood? You wouldn't have to worry about a career, a car payment, rent or taxes. You wouldn't have to worry about securing your future or carrying the burden of your regrets from the past. Your responsibilities would be limited in scope to things like cleaning your room, taking out the trash or mowing the lawn.

This dream is common amongst most adults. We revere youth. Consider our clichés "Youth is wasted on the young"; "If I only knew then what I know now," "Hind sight is 20/20," "He's just a big kid."

Look at our literature and movies. Arguably the most popular children's story ever told is about an ageless child from a place called Never Never Land, where kids can be kids forever. One of the most popular movies in the last 20 years is "Big" with Tom Hanks. It tells the story of a young boy that makes a wish to be older. His wish is granted and hilarity ensues, but by the end of the movie, the main character gets tired of being an adult and returns to being a boy.

While most of us can only dream of being young again, Randy actually lives it. He has been given the gift of an eternal childhood. To put it simply, Randy never really matured past the mental age of about eight. That's not to say that in all aspects, he is exactly like an eight year old boy, but there are many.

Remember being eight years old? It was a great age. You weren't a baby that needed constant attention, but you weren't a teenager struggling for complete autonomy. You were big enough to play outside by yourself, but too young to really go anywhere outside your immediate neighborhood. You could enjoy the sweet pain of a puppy love crush, but were too young to comprehend the commitment and sacrifice of a real relationship. You had Saturday morning cartoons, and Saturday afternoon matinees, Rated G. Your imagination was as close to reality as it would ever be.

Today, Randy is physically 48 years old, yet every Saturday morning he can be found, in his *jammies,* with a bowl of cereal, watching cartoons. His imagination is still king.

If you were to walk into his bedroom you would see what seems like a child's bedroom. There is a wooden toy train on his dresser and a Power Ranger's doll in the corner. The shelves in his room are filled with videos of Snow White, The Lion King, Mary Poppins, Superman and the like.

Yet something isn't quite right. There are no dirty socks lying on the floor. No half eaten cookie behind the dresser. No crayon marks on the walls. No Kool-Aid stain on the carpet. It's too clean to be a kid's room.

His clothes are hung neatly in the closet; Pants on one side shirts on the other, each one half inch apart. His underwear is folded and arranged strategically alongside tightly-rolled socks in his top dresser drawer. The other giveaway is the tall four-post queen-sized bed.

See, what really separates Randy from the typical eight year-old is about 37 years of extra living experience. Unlike most eight year olds, Randy is meticulous and very well organized. He keeps a schedule and holds down two jobs.

Not everything about being eight was great. Remember how slowly time went by when you were eight and waiting for something? Two weeks could seem like an eternity. And it was always two weeks. Two weeks until the new must see movie was released, two weeks until your big birthday party, two weeks until summer vacation. Patience sucked.

Remember asking a grown up to explain something to you and the stock answer was, "You'll understand when you are older?" Remember desperately wanting to be older—so much so that we stated our age in fractions? "I'm eight … *and a half!*" That half year can be critical in determining social pecking order. Adults do it to, only in reverse. "This is the 12th anniversary of my 29th birthday."

In my opinion, one of the greatest ironies of human existence is that the young want to be old and the old want to be young.

This is the paradox in which Randy finds himself. He is young and old at the same time. In many ways he has the best of both worlds, in some ways he has the frustrations of both. Regardless, this dichotomy is the basis for the unique relationship I have shared with the one man who has been a big brother, a twin, and little brother to me.

Big Brother

When I was born, Randy was almost seven years old. By the time I was out of diapers, he was ten and was everything a kid could want in a big brother.

To me, he was *smart*. Mom had finally gotten him into the mainstream public schools and he was thriving. In those days, most kids learned the ABC's around the age of five which was first grade or at the earliest, kindergarten. Randy was ten but I didn't know he was behind. He would come home from school and teach me what he was learning. I was three when I first learned my ABC's thanks to my brother, the professor. It was good for Randy too, because by teaching me, he forced himself to really retain what he was learning in school. It has been my experience that the best way to really learn something is to teach it. Randy also had the patience to teach me that no one else had. My earliest childhood memory is sitting with my big brother writing big A's and little a's for hours.

Today, children are learning much more at an early age. Anyone with a young child today is probably familiar with the Baby Einstein Series of videos by Julie Clark. These videos expose toddlers and even infants to the alphabet, shapes, colors, animals, music, you name it. My son, Jackson, could recite the entire alphabet and knew all the prominent shapes and colors by the time he was 18 months old, thanks in large part to Ms. Clark's videos. In a strange way, Randy was a vanguard. He was my Baby Einstein.

Like most big brothers, Randy was also my protector. I always felt safe when I was around him. We shared a room until I was in high school. I had the top bunk and he had the bottom bunk. Whenever there was a thunderstorm, I would climb down to the bottom bunk. He would wrap his arms around me and the thunder wouldn't matter. When we watched TV, Randy's favorite spot was in a brown bean bag chair. My favorite spot was in his lap. I was like his dog. When he left for school in the morning I would watch him walk down the street with my sister, lunch boxes in hand. In the afternoon I'd stare out the kitchen window waiting to see him turn the corner onto our street, and then I would run out to greet him.

One morning, my Mom got a phone call from a lady that lived at the corner. She said she had seen me turning the corner with what looked like a silverware basket from the dishwasher. When Mom caught me, I told her that I wanted to go to school and see Randy. The silverware basket was my make believe lunch box.

One summer, Dad took the family to Myrtle Beach, South Carolina on vacation. I was making castles in the sand and some older kids kept kicking them down. Randy saw this and rushed to my rescue. He ran up and without warning pushed the biggest kid down then grabbed my arm and we took off running. The other kids chased us. Randy was fast but he never let me fall behind. The chase ended abruptly when they saw us wrapped around our Dad's legs.

Randy was much bigger than the kid he pushed. Not long after, the kid's Dad came over and said angrily, "Keep that retard away from my son." Much to my surprise, Dad was cool and calm. He could have defended Randy and told that man that his kid was a bully and had it coming to him. I wanted Dad to punch the guy in the nose. Instead, he diplomatically diffused the situation. Dad understood that people react irrationally out of fear to what they don't understand.

Dad scolded us and said that the next time something like that happens, to just walk away. He said, "Fighting is not the answer. It takes a bigger man to walk away from a fight, than it does to stay and fight like an animal."

Keep in mind, Dad was a tough guy. This wisdom was coming from a man that grew up in a poor neighborhood, without a father or other positive male role model. He labored in the apple orchards as a kid and played smash mouth football in high school and college at a time when padding was limited and helmets were optional. He was a fighter pilot who courted death on a daily basis by strapping himself to a rocket loaded with bombs and flying faster than the speed of sound. He was a soldier who had been to war, had been shot down behind enemy lines and fought his way out. He was fearless and no one could ever call this man a coward. Yet he was telling us to just walk away. Why? I wouldn't figure out the answer until years later.

With the exception of this one incident, Randy was never violent. He didn't mean to hurt that other kid. He just wanted to get them away from me.

It was the only time I've ever seen Randy physically harm anyone. Anyone other than me I should say, but that's what brothers, especially twins, do.

Twins

By the time I was eight years old, I had somewhat caught up with my brother. Randy and I were like twins. It has been said that there is a special bond between twins. They seem to know what each other is thinking. They can finish each other's sentences. They seem to sense when the other is in trouble and so on. Well, that wasn't really the case with Randy and me, but it was close.

We didn't look anything like each other. Even fraternal twins have certain similar characteristics. Because of the common physical traits related to Down Syndrome, one could hardly tell we were even related. Besides, he was fifteen years old and much bigger than I. But we did everything together.

Before, I had been the kid brother that always tagged along. Something most big brothers get tired of, but not Randy. He was a great big brother. The only time I didn't get to go with him was when he went to Boy Scout troop meetings. *He was a better big brother than I would one day be.*

For now, we were inseparable. We liked all the same things; comic books, toys, TV shows. We would ride our bikes everywhere together.

He was better than a twin because of his size. In the summer, we would go to the community pool. Randy is a great swimmer and to this day still swims 60 laps in the pool every day for exercise. Back then we would do what we called "push ups." Randy would go under water and I would sit on his shoulders. He would then stand up and launch me into the air like a catapult and I would come splashing down. We would do this for hours. Not many big brothers would do this for as long as Randy did.

Another one of our favorite things to do was build a little bike ramp out of cinderblocks and a piece of plywood. He could carry two cinder blocks instead of one. We would pretend we were Evil Knievel and would jump over just about anything we could find.

We were the best of friends yet we were also *brothers* and like all brothers, we had the occasional disagreement. Actually we fought like crazy. We would fight over anything; who had to rake the lawn or do the dishes. We fought over who got to ride in the *front* seat of the car. We fought over who got the bigger slice of cake. Mom solved this one ingeniously. One of us would cut the cake and the other would choose. You better believe that each piece of cake from then on was halved with scientific precision.

Our fights rarely got physical, probably because Randy was twice my size, but also because Randy just didn't have violence in him. Most of our fights were screaming matches with the occasional punch on the arm or the dreaded "foobuh." A "foobuh" was a "foot to the butt."

I vividly remember the last time we physically fought. It was a rainy summer day and the community pool was closed so we played most of the day inside. What had started as a harmless pillow fight escalated to a wrestling match. Randy quickly pinned me down and wouldn't let me up which just made me mad. When he finally let me up, I grabbed a plastic whiffle ball bat and chased him around the house. Randy ran out the front door and slipped on the wet lawn and broke his leg. I got in a lot of trouble for that. Randy was in a cast for six weeks and couldn't go swimming for the rest of the summer. I felt so bad that I didn't go to the pool either. I sat in the house with him and played games. It was during this time that we came up with our "secret hand shake" that we still do to this day.

This time would also mark the beginning of the end of our relationship as twins. The scolding I received from Mom and Dad was fortified with instructions that I should look after Randy. I began to comprehend some meaning behind the term "special" brother. Before then, this term just meant he was different. I never wanted to see my brother hurt again. From then on, I slipped into the role of protector and gradually became the big brother.

Little Brother

With each passing summer, we did fewer and fewer pushups, partly because I was getting too big for Randy to lift me out of the water and partly because I had grown out of the shallow end of the pool where most of the younger kids played. I spent my pool time with the other hormonally challenged teenage boys at the diving boards, doing back flips to impress the girls who couldn't care less. Standing on that board I could see my big brother, in the shallow end, playing pushups with the other eight year olds. He always waved at me and I always waved back.

One time I couldn't find my bathing suit so I just wore a pair of white tennis shorts to the pool. Little did I know, these shorts when wet, were as transparent as a campaign promise. Randy was kind enough to point this out to everyone who hadn't already noticed. From the shallow end he raised his hand with his thumb and fore finger about an inch apart and shouted, "There's my LITTLE brother Bobby." The place erupted in laughter and I cursed the cold water that day.

There was definitely a gap widening in our relationship. In the years to come when we would go somewhere together, Mom would admonish me to take good care of Randy thus putting me in a position of authority over him. Randy even began to refer to me as his big brother. Randy and I had what we called "Buddy-Buddy Days." They were reserved for him and me to do anything we wanted together. Usually we'd go to lunch and then go to an afternoon movie, or the skating rink, or the mall, or the bowling alley, etc. It was a time when Randy got my undivided attention.

My teenage years were pretty typical of the late 70's and early 80's. Skating rinks, gym dances and the mall were the center of my social life. On most occasions, as I was leaving the house for one of these destinations, Randy would be at the door asking if he could come with me. Like most big brothers, I didn't want him tagging along. Not because I was ashamed or embarrassed that I had a Down Syndrome brother. That has never been the case. But primarily because Randy was a responsibility and responsibility is not necessarily a teenager's strong point. Besides, we had our Buddy-Buddy Days together and this was my time to be with my friends and not have to worry about anyone else.

It was hard for me to say no to Randy. Quite often I would say no, and then as I was driving away I would look back and see his sad face pressed against the kitchen window watching me go; much like I used to do when I was younger as he went off to school. Invariably I would turn around. He'd come running out of the house with the biggest smile on his face and we'd head off together.

Wherever we went, I had to make sure he didn't wander off. There have been a few times when I would hear my name over the loud speaker at the mall instructing me to meet my "party" at the information desk.

Randy also waits until the very last second to tell you he has to go to the bathroom. When he has to go, he has to go immediately. This can be a problem if you have to search for a bathroom. From time to time our nights would be cut short by "accidents."

Randy wasn't just a responsibility though. He got along well with all my friends. If I'm going to be honest in telling this story I'll have to say that there were selfish reasons to have him around also. I got attention for having him with me, especially from girls. Girls loved Randy. When I saw a pretty girl, that I didn't know I would send Randy over to introduce himself. He is such a charmer. He would use the cheesy pick up lines like, "Gee you look beautiful tonight," or "You have beautiful eyes." If I had said those things, they would have seen right through me and brushed me off with the flip of the hair, but coming from Randy these lines worked. I would then come over and Randy would introduce me. I was perceived as being safe and trustworthy for taking care of him. This was how I met my high school sweetheart.

Another benefit of having Randy around was that he gave me an excuse not to succumb to peer pressure. Whenever my friends wanted to do something that I didn't feel right about doing, I could always back out gracefully because I had Randy with me. However, sometimes when I *wanted* to do something crazy that I knew I shouldn't, Randy would keep me from doing it simply because Randy is incapable of keeping a secret. I would tell him explicitly not to tell Mom and Dad that we threw eggs at the mayor's house. When we got home Mom and Dad would ask what we did and Randy would say, "Bobby told me not to tell you."

I didn't always take Randy with me and there were more than a few times that I wished I had.

When I went off to college, Randy was quite distraught. He called me every day for the first month. Back then, there were no cell phones and long distance calls were expensive. So we worked out a schedule when he could call and I would do my best to be in the dorm at that time. We picked Saturday mornings at 11:00 AM.

I looked forward to our calls and Randy was always called on time. One Saturday morning towards the end of my first semester, I waited for his call but it never came. I got a little worried so I called home and Mom answered. She told me that Randy had gone to lunch and a movie with a guy named Troy Landavazo. Troy was a junior in high school and worked with Randy at the Air Force Base Officer's Club bussing tables. Mom said he was really nice and that he had been taking Randy out regularly. Admittedly I was jealous. I didn't like the fact that someone else was having a Buddy-Buddy Day with *my* brother.

I called back later that afternoon to talk to Randy. I asked him about Troy and he told me all of the things they were doing together. Troy had been taking him bowling and to movies, etc. He even took Randy with him when he went on dates. I asked Randy if he thought of Troy like a brother. Randy replied, "He's better than a brother."

My heart sank. I couldn't blame him though. I was the one who left, but that didn't make me feel any better about it.

Two weeks later, my first semester was over and I drove home for Christmas break. I had to meet this Troy guy. Surely he couldn't be as good as Mom and Randy made him out to be. There had to be a dark side of him somewhere. On the drive home I conjured up malicious theories in my head. I thought, they can't see through him but I can. I figured at the very least he was probably using Randy to get girls, *like I had done.*

My parents had a welcome home party for me that night. Troy was there. We hung out together most of the night. I found nothing to validate my petty fears. The next day, Troy and I took Randy bowling and we all had a great time. The three of us spent most of the Christmas vacation together. Troy and I became the best of friends.

The next year, Troy's parents moved away but Troy wanted to finish high school where he started. He moved in with my parents, in my room no less, and stayed until graduation. He continued to take Randy with him the whole time. Troy became part of our family. We call each other "Brothers From Another Mother."

Today, Troy lives with his wife Kammy and son Nico in New Mexico. Randy flies out there every year for at least a one-week visit. Troy and Kammy are also the Godparents to my son Jackson.

I feel very blessed to have had the unique experience of having a big brother, a twin, and a little brother all in one person. He has also been my teacher, my protector and now my muse. However, the story doesn't end here. Our unique relationship would evolve one more time into something even more priceless.

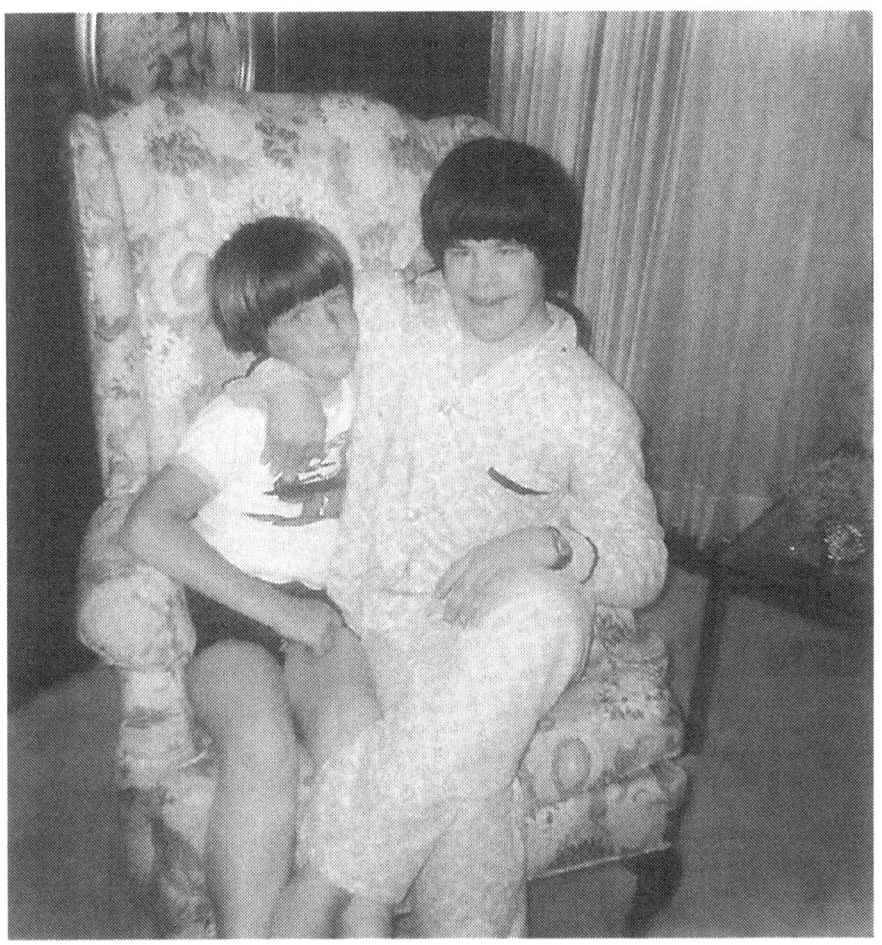

Randy and Opey

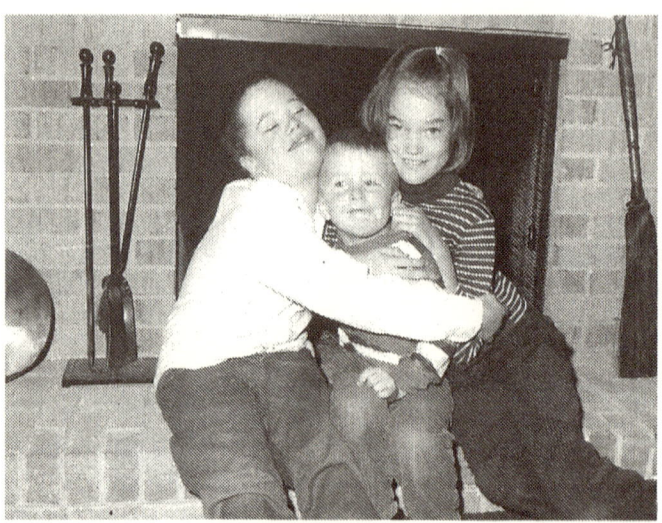

Randy, Opey, and Robin

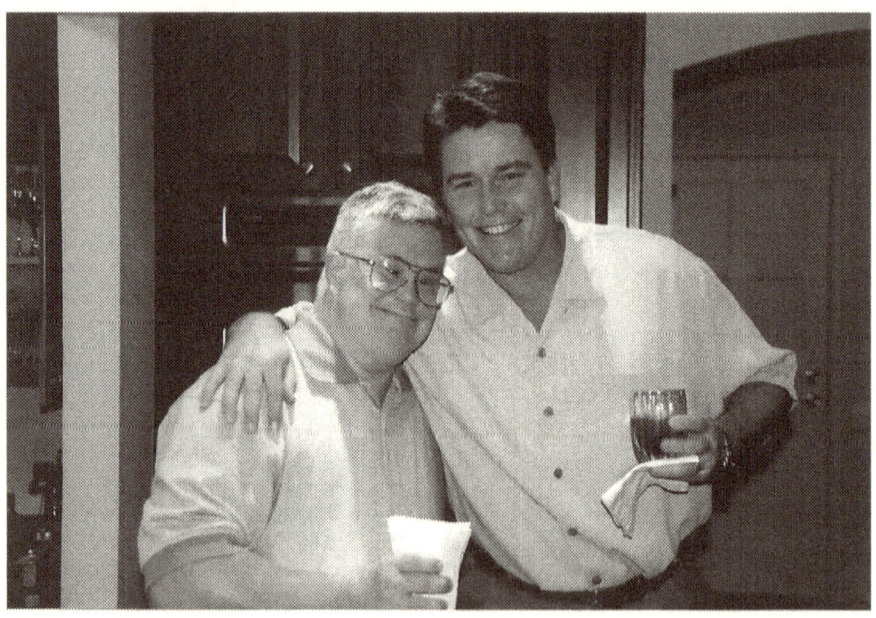

Randy and Opey Cocktail Hour

7

Phones in Heaven

March 7, 1998, would have been Dad's 65th birthday. Seven years earlier, during his retirement physical, he was diagnosed with prostate cancer. The day after his retirement, he had surgery followed by radiation treatment. Everything seemed fine. I was living in Los Angeles at the time and I remember my Mom calling me from his hospital room to tell me that all went well. She was disappointed that I hadn't called. Truthfully it never crossed my mind that he would be anything *but* OK. Nothing could beat my Dad; not war, not cancer, not even my teenage years although I'm sure I came close.

Mom and Dad had spent 36 years in the Air Force. Mandatory retirement for an Air Force officer is 35 years, but the first Gulf war came around right when Dad's 35 years were up. Since Dad was the Commander of TAC, that meant that he was in charge of all the fighter pilots and the planning of the initial air war over Iraq. He leaving now would be like changing head coaches just before the Super Bowl so he was asked to stay on until the war was over. Not being one to leave a job undone, Dad agreed. His retirement would have to wait.

Mom and Dad had simple plans for their retirement. They wanted to build their dream home on a bay somewhere in sunny Florida and live their remaining days playing golf, going fishing and having dinner parties with their friends. Travel was out of the question. They had spent the last six years of their career traveling to all corners of the globe. Dad was planning on working for a defense contractor for a couple of years. Retired Four Star General's are sought after in the civilian defense business. Because of his health, he decided not to take a full time job and only worked on a consulting basis.

Instead, he threw himself into building their home. But that did not prove to be any less stressful. After two years of dishonest subcontractors and Hurricane

Opal, their dream home was finally finished and they moved in. Seven months later his cancer came out of remission and within six weeks it was all over.

Mom, my sister Robin and I were at his side holding his hands as he lay in his bed at home. He had slipped into a coma a day earlier. Hospice had given him a morphine pump so we were relatively certain he wasn't in any pain. At 4:28 PM on May 22, 1998, he took one last deep breath, clenched our hands then opened his eyes and looked at Mom and mouthed the words, "I love you Jeanie." He then slowly slipped into the hereafter.

Randy wasn't in the room at the time of Dad's death. He couldn't handle what was happening. As hard as this was for us, it was even harder on Randy. In all my years with him I had never seen my brother cry from emotion. Oh sure, he cried when he stubbed his toe or skinned his knee as a child, but never from emotion. On this day, he wailed. He cried so much, his shirt was drenched. We tried to comfort him, but he wouldn't let anyone near him. He just shut his door and cried and cried and cried.

This was Randy's first real experience with death. He had seen people die on TV, but that was make believe, this was real. It would be a long time before Randy was back to his jovial self. It was nine and a half months before he set foot again in Mom and Dad's bedroom.

When the frenzy of the funeral subsided, Mom was left in the house without her husband of 40 years. She was alone for the first time in her life. But she wasn't. She still had a purpose. My sister and I were grown and away, but Randy was still there. He needed her and she needed him. He kept her going through the roughest time in her life and he's still there. They golf together, take their pontoon boat out on the lake, go bowling and out to dinner. One of Randy's gifts to Mom was that he spared her the desperate loneliness of a widow and gave her a reason to continue living. They also had the support and friendship of great friends, Chuck and Mary Jo Horner. Dad and Chuck were Air Force Generals. They are neighbors to Mom and Randy and are close, caring, and supportive friends.

March 7th 1998, Dad's Birthday. Breakfast was ready and we called for Randy but he didn't come. I went to his room but he wasn't there. It wasn't like Randy to miss a meal. We finally found him standing at the edge of the bed where Dad had died.

He looked up at Mom and me and asked with all sincerity, "Do they have phones in heaven?"

For some reason, Birthdays are huge for Randy. He loves a birthday party more than anything. I think maybe it's because birthday parties are always a celebration. There's never really anyone sad or angry at one another. Randy, like most people with Down Syndrome, thrive on happiness and joy. It's a state where they always want to be. Not unlike the rest of us, only we find ways to sabotage ourselves from constantly being in this state. Most people will find reasons to be unhappy. Our job is boring; we aren't making enough money; it's too cold or too hot outside, are some of the things we use as excuses to not being happy.

I have a newspaper clipping of a Family Circus cartoon on my desk. I think it pretty much sums up the way in which most people with Down Syndrome look at life. The cartoon depicts the four seasons. The first picture is Spring and it's raining and the kid is in his rain coat and boots, splashing gleefully in puddles on his way home from school. The second picture is Summer and the kid is cheerfully making sand castles at the beach. The third is Fall and the kid is playing joyfully through a big pile of leaves. The fourth is Winter and the kids are all bundled up and excitedly sledding down a hill. The caption reads, "There is no such thing as bad weather, only different kinds of good weather."

We all have the ability to choose our moods regardless of the situation in which we find ourselves. Luckily for Randy, his choices are automatic. He doesn't have to think about how he feels. He has been given the gift of choosing happiness at every turn without effort; a feat even the best self-help guru cannot match.

So on this somber morning, the first birthday since our father's death, Randy has made his choice. Rather than sulk or cry or feel sorry for ourselves for our loss, he wants to call his Dad in Heaven to wish him happy birthday.

When we told him that there were no phones in heaven he didn't get upset or discouraged, he simply went to the kitchen table and ate his breakfast. We didn't know it at the time but Randy made another choice at that moment; choice not unlike the one Mom and Dad made when they first learned of Randy's condition. Mom and Dad knew that no matter what they did, Randy would always have Down Syndrome, but that didn't stop them from trying to better his life. Randy also knew that no matter how many numbers he dialed, there were no phones in heaven, but that wasn't going to stop him from trying to find another way.

That evening we decided to go to dinner to celebrate our Dad's life. On the way to the restaurant, Randy asked us to stop at the Albertson's supermarket where he worked. We asked him why but he wouldn't say. He was insistent, we had to stop now.

Randy and I went into the store and he headed straight to the party supplies section. Several minutes later we returned to the car with three white helium filled balloons. After all, what's a birthday party without balloons? He was determined to make this a jovial affair.

We were seated at a table for four at one of Dad's favorite Italian restaurants. Randy tied the balloons to the empty chair where Dad should have been sitting. Mom struggled to hold back the tears. The mood was somber until Randy stood up and announced that he had to go to the bathroom. Usually one would not make such an announcement in a voice that could be heard beyond the table. However, Randy is not quite adept at such social subtleties. Mom and I could not help but chuckle.

Randy was in the bathroom for a long time. Just as I was about to go check on him he came out. Mom and I watched in disbelief as he apologetically stated to each table along the way, "Sorry I took so long, I've got diarrhea."

Later we had a little talk with Randy.

The mood was considerably less somber from then until the time the check came.

When the waitress returned with the credit card slip, Randy reached for it. He wanted to sign just like Dad always did. Mom let him sign the check, not the actual credit card slip, and we thanked him for buying us dinner. As kids we would compete to be the first to thank Dad for taking us out to dinner. Now

Randy was being thanked and in his mind it must have been a symbolic passing of the torch. To this day, he insists on signing the check.

After he signed the check Mom, reached for the pen and Randy held back.

"Wait just a second Mom," he said.

He took one of the balloons off of *Dad's* chair and carefully wrote the following on it.

"Dear Dad, Happy Birthday. I miss you. Love, Your Son, Randy Russ"

Randy handed us the other balloons and the pen then said, "Since there are no phones in heaven, I thought we'd send him a birthday card."

Mom and I wrote our own personal messages, and then the three of us went outside, stood in the parking lot, and mailed the balloons to heaven.

The next morning at the breakfast table Randy asked, "Do you think Dad got the message by now?"

Yes Randy, I'm sure he did. *And so did we.*

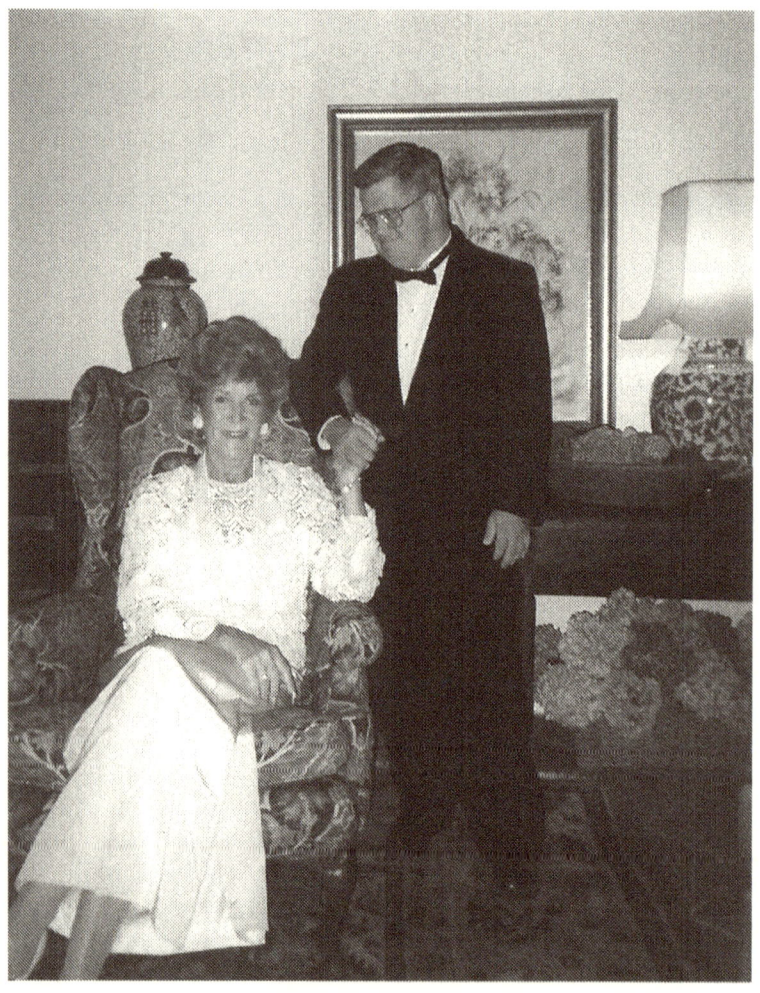

Mom and Randy

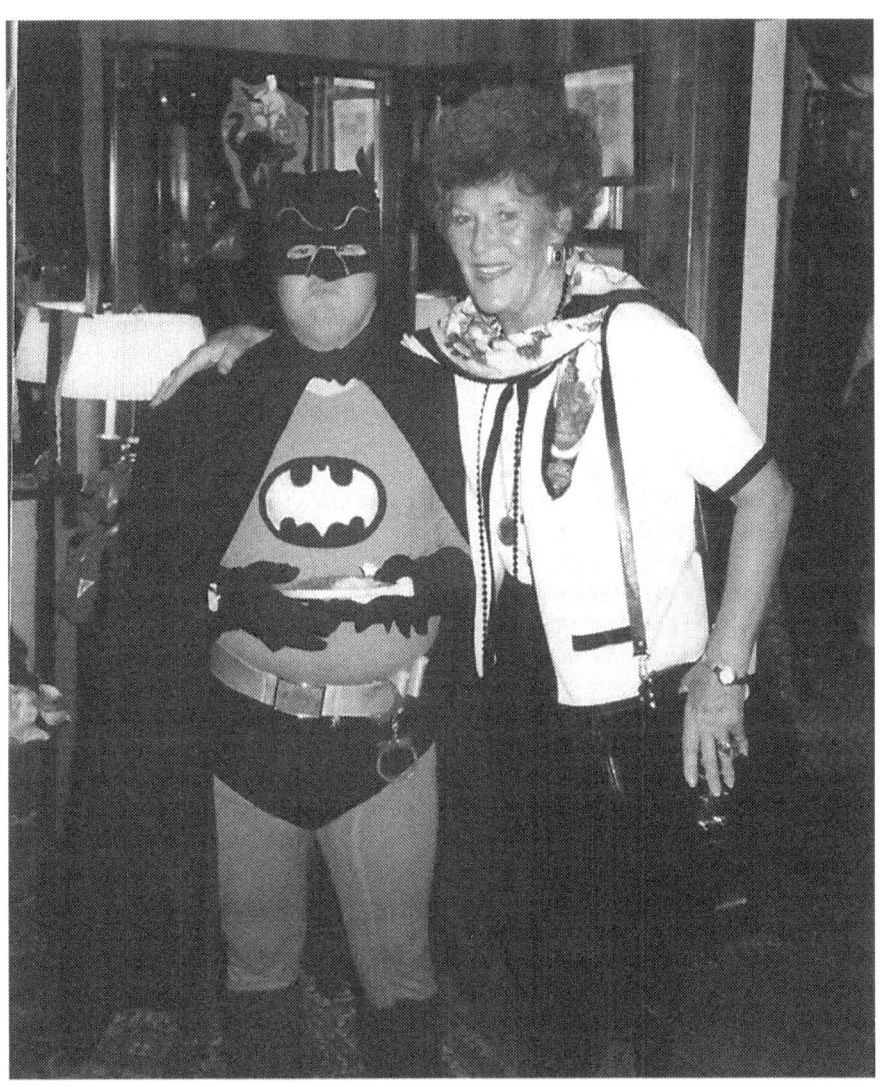

Happy Halloween—Randy and Mom

8

... And a Son

Angela and I had been married for only six months when she called me in to the bathroom to take the test. Why they actually put directions on those things I'll never know. It's quite simple really, if the test strip turns purple then you start paying attention to diaper commercials. However, the gravity of the situation somehow forces you to read the directions anyway.

For as long as I can remember, I've wanted to be a dad. My relationship with my dad was about as good as it could be. He was my hero and I was his name sake.

"Do you know what the first words out of Dad's mouth were when you were born?" Mom used to ask.

It's one of those questions that mom's ask not because they think you don't know the answer, but because they want to tell you.

"He's going to mow my lawn?" I always reply. She's never amused.

"He's exactly what I wanted," is what he actually said.

He was a great dad. We did all the typical father-son activities. We played catch and went fishing. He taught me how to wield a wrench, first on my bike, then on the lawn mower and eventually on the 'Stang'. The 'Stang' was little more than the frame and right front fender of a 1966 Ford Mustang convertible when Dad first pulled it out of a junk yard. We worked on it together until it was restored to its original brilliance—candy apple red with a shiny black interior. He used to tell me that he bought it because it was made the same year I was born and so that one day I would own a car as old as me. For many years he drove that car and it became his trademark.

Dad set high standards of behavior and was firm in enforcing them. Yet he was kind, forgiving and patient. We were never physically punished. Instead, he would make us go to our room and think about our discretions. We weren't allowed out until we could explain to him exactly what we had done wrong and why we chose to do it. Placing blame on others or making excuses out of circumstances only extended our sentence. He stressed personal responsibility and integrity above all else.

The older I got, the more I would think about how I was going to get out of my room *before* I did something suspect. I would actually rehearse my speech to Dad in my head. More often than not, I would come to the conclusion that there was just no way I was going to get out without a complete confession. My decisions were then based on whether or not I was willing to accept the consequences of my actions. Quite simply, if the consequences outweighed the fun of doing something, then I didn't do it; otherwise, I did it and took my lumps.

I guess having a great dad makes you want to be one. This desire was never stronger in me than in the months following my dad's death. I had lost that relationship and I desperately wanted it back. So as my wife and I left that bathroom with the *purple* test strip in hand, I was elated. I was finally going to be a dad and I was going to be as much like my dad as possible.

We spent the next eight weeks considering baby names and planning to remodel our guest room into a nursery. Unfortunately, no name would get the job and the guest room would remain still. Ultimately, three more miscarriages would follow.

These were tough times for us, but I was given an unexpected blessing to help me get through them. This is where the unique relationship with my three-in-one brother took its final turn.

During his career, Dad was extremely busy. He was out of the house by 5:30 in the morning and got home around 6:00 at night. He traveled extensively. He didn't make it to every little league game or my sister's recitals, but he always found a way to make it to the important ones. I'm certain he missed us as much, if not more, than we missed him.

When most successful people retire, they look back on their lives and wonder if they should have spent more time with their families. Inevitably they will find times when they wish they had spent more time with their kids. I'm sure this was the case with my father as well. However, Dad was given a blessing that he couldn't have thought of forty years earlier. It was the blessing of a second chance at fatherhood.

One of Randy's gifts to our Dad was the second chance at fatherhood. My sister and I were grown and gone when Dad retired. Randy was still there, a loving eight year old with a few grey hairs. Dad spent his final years taking Randy fishing, to ball games, movies, the zoo and even Disney World. He remarked to Mom several times, "What would we do if we didn't have Randy? Then followed it up with, "I wouldn't change him even if I could."

Randy finally got the dedicated, consistent, quality time with Dad we had all wanted years ago. He just waited it out and it came.

So when Dad died, Randy took it exceptionally hard. He and Dad had grown so much closer in those final years. Just as I was missing the father-son relationship, so was Randy. And so it happened that the man that had been three different brothers to me became my son.

The change was subtle at first. Randy and I were on a Buddy-Buddy Day and I asked him if he liked his new job at Albertson's supermarket. He replied, "Yes sir." Sir? That was a moniker reserved only for Dad. I didn't think much of it at the time, but I did tell Mom later that day and we had a good laugh.

About a week later, Mom asked if I would pick Randy up from work. It was a beautiful day so I pulled the 'Stang' out of my garage and put the top down. For many years I rode shotgun in that car. Things looked and felt different from where I sat now. The sweetness of my new perspective was tainted slightly by the bitterness of the reason why.

Randy's face lit up when he saw me pull up in that majestic car. My pride betrayed any sense of cool I tried to portray. We ended up driving around for a while. He then said, "Are you proud of me?" Randy was always seeking Dads approval as were the rest of us and here he was now seeking mine.

I embraced my new found position. It was easy and familiar. It was make believe—for real. Since my wife and I had no children, Randy filled the void in me to be a father, and not just *any* father but OUR father. Randy would frequently remark how I looked and sounded like Dad. I've been accused of being a pretty good mimic and I have to admit that at times I would put on my "Dad" voice just to elicit such a response.

From time to time, Mom would have to go out of town for a reunion or a funeral, sometimes both. I was charged with taking care of Randy during these times. So my wife and I converted the empty nursery to a bedroom for Randy, complete with TV, VCR and CD player for his Partridge Family recordings. When Randy stays with us we try to make the environment as close to home as possible. He has the same chores, mainly emptying the dishwasher and taking out the trash. Since Randy likes to follow a schedule we keep pretty close to his. Breakfast at 8:00 AM, lunch at 1:00 PM, cocktail (diet coke) at 5 PM, Partridge Family concert at 5:30 PM, dinner at 7:00 PM, dessert at 9:00 PM, and finally prayers and bedtime at 11:00 PM. Mom is never out of town for more than a week so I try to fit in at least one Buddy Buddy Day when he's with us.

I always looked forward to Randy staying with us. For a while, the fatherhood void in me that he was filling was enough. Then one day our phone rang and it was an adoption lawyer. A friend of ours, Jack Krayniak, referred her to us. She said there was a baby to be born in a couple of months and from what Jack had told her about us, we had a good chance of adopting. Angela and I were ecstatic and we quickly took care of all the legal adoption requirements.

Two weeks before the due date, Randy and I were getting ready for a Buddy Buddy Day when the phone rang. The baby was coming two weeks early and I had to get to the hospital. I looked at Randy and said, "I can't take you to lunch today Randy."

His chin fell to his chest. "Why not?" he mumbled.

I hated to disappoint him but this was serious and I had to go. I took his face in my hands and said, "Because my son is being born."

What he said next shocked me. Randy knew we were adopting a baby boy but I never knew how that affected him. He took my hands from his face and with a look like I had just stabbed him in the back said, "But I'm your son."

It hit me at that moment that Randy would forever more be my son. And while I have a son of my own now, and the desire to be a father has been fulfilled, I know that Randy will always have that longing for that special father-son relationship, and I will always oblige.

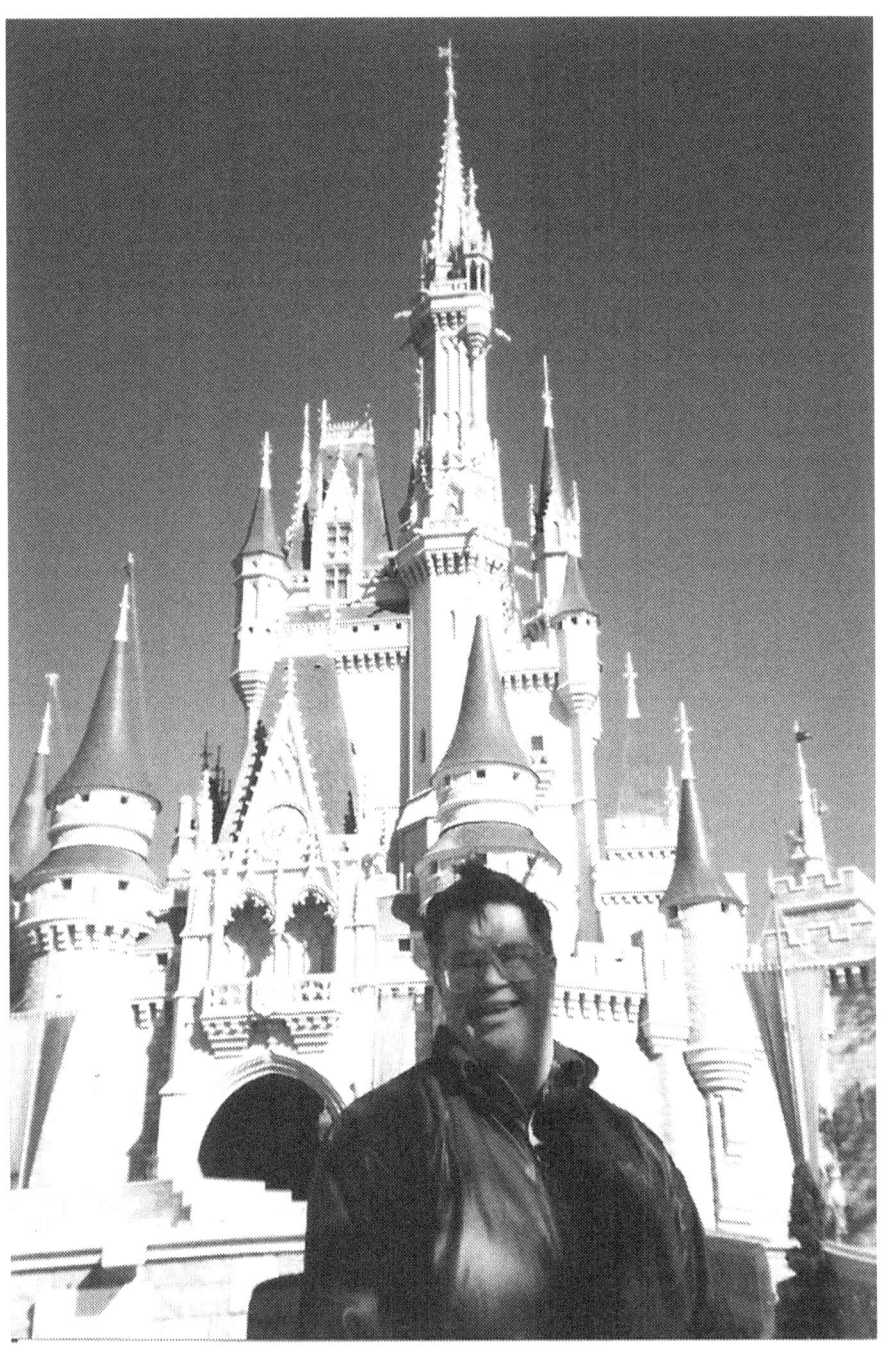

Randy's favorite place—the Castle (Feb 96)

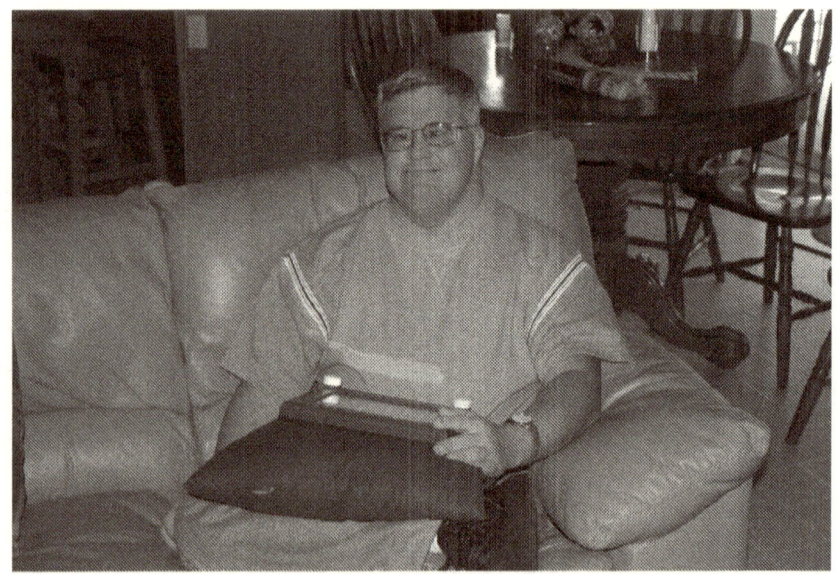

Randy loves his etch-a-sketch

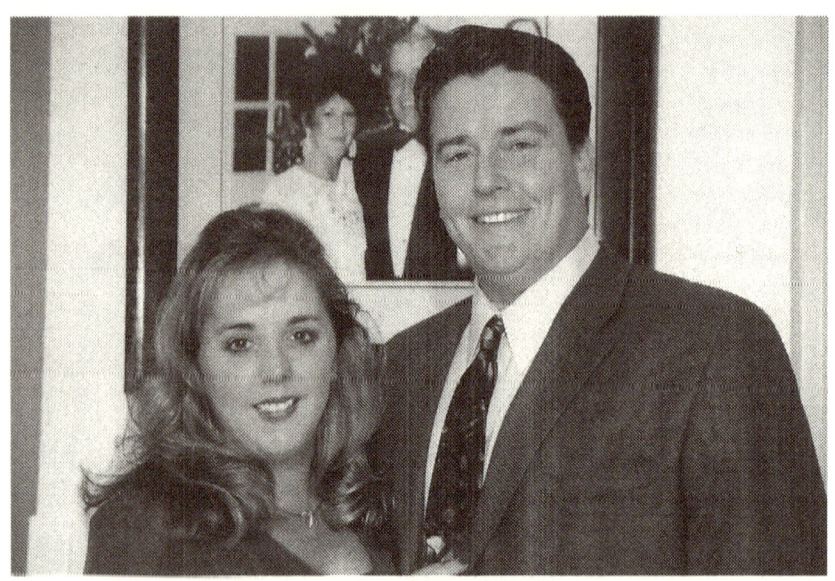

Opey and Angela

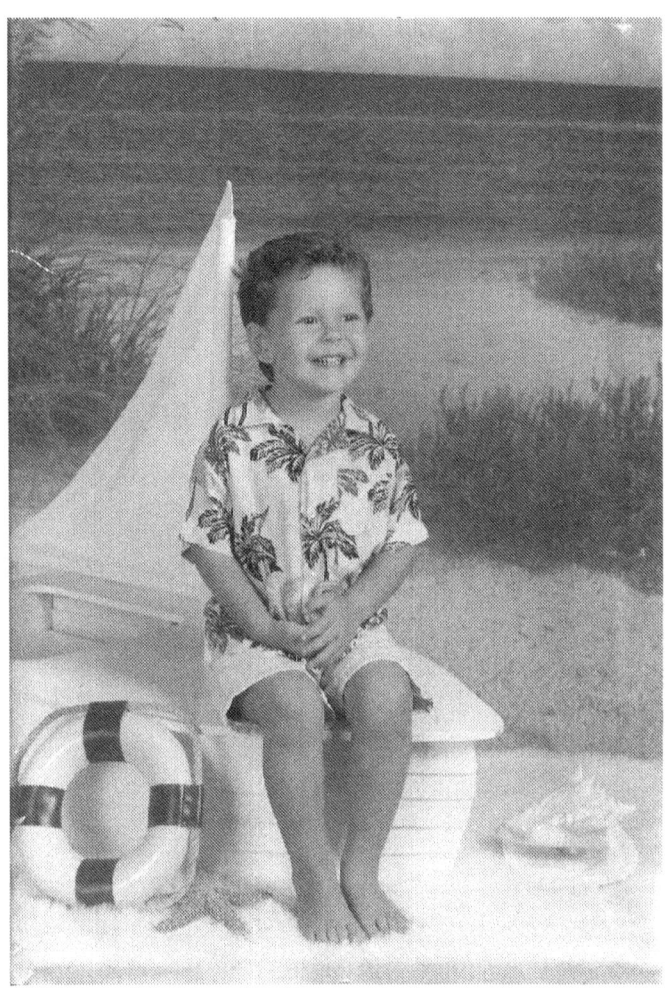

My son Jackson

9

Randy's Angels

Someone once said it's not who you love or how you love but that you love. Other than his mother and sister, Randy has had several significant women in his life; Barbara, Gail, and the Angels from Destin.

Barbara

Randy and Barbara met at the officers' club pool on Seymour Johnson Air Force Base in the summer of 1976. She was a 17 year old beauty queen and the favorite life guard of all the kids; the quintessential all-American girl next door.

Barbara took to Randy immediately. She would take him out dining and to movies and parties with her friends. Randy was clearly smitten with her. She frequently stopped by our home un-announced just to spend a little time with Randy. If we had company at the house, Randy would put his arm around her and introduce her as his "girlfriend." She always played along.

The night of her senior prom, she stopped by the house after the dance to see Randy. Mom recalls that she and Dad asked her all about the prom. Being humble, she downplayed the evening, never telling them she was elected prom queen.

Barbara was Randy's first love. He would day dream of marrying her and having a house of their own. Like most first loves, it wouldn't last. Barbara would eventually go off to college where she graduated magna cum laude from Appalachian State University then got her law degree from the University of North Carolina. They would talk on the phone from time to time and all the while, Randy never stopped calling her his "girlfriend."

Then one day Barbara called and told Randy she was getting married. In typical Randy fashion he replied, "I'm so happy for you!" and he meant it.

Barbara invited Randy to the wedding and he and Mom attended. To this day, Randy keeps a photo of him and Barbara on the dresser in his room. A sweet reminder of his first love.

Gail

When Dad was stationed at the Pentagon in the late 70's and early 80's, Randy met Gail at a social activity sponsored by the local Association of Retarded Citizens (ARC). Though not a person with Down Syndrome, Gail had some developmental disabilities, but Randy saw only her beauty. Gail was in her mid 20's and she simply adored Randy. She often remarked how handsome he looked in his glasses.

They would plan frequent dates, usually to dinner and a movie. Mom would play chauffer and chaperone. In her compassionate wisdom, Mom realized that it couldn't be considered a real date if she sat with them so she would wait in the lounge or somewhere out of sight. On one occasion, Mom decided to check up on them and noticed that there were five orders of guacamole on the table. The waitress thought she could pad the check easily on this table. Mom confronted her and eventually had the manager take the four extra orders off the check. From that moment on, Mom always kept a safe distance on their dates and would instruct the manager to bring her the check. If everything looked ok, she would pay it then have the receipt delivered to the table. Randy took pride in thinking he was paying the bill so he would sign the receipt as if he were actually signing a credit card slip.

As time went by, their relationship blossomed. They would talk on the phone almost nightly, eagerly making plans for their next date. When the annual weekend retreat, sponsored by the local ARC came around, they were excited, to say the least. And then it happened. On the bus heading for the retreat, Gail turned to Randy and said, "Randy, would you like to kiss me?"

Most people have their first kiss in their early teens. I remember mine like it was yesterday. I was twelve and I kissed a girl in an empty dugout at the little league baseball field. My heart nearly leapt out of my chest and I floated on air for days.

I can only imagine what this moment must have been like for Randy. He was 30 years old and about to get his first real kiss. To this day if you ask Randy what his answer to Gail's question was he says with a bashful grin, "I said, I accept"

And they kissed.

When the kiss was over, Gail said to Randy that he kissed like Scott Baio (Chachi) and he replied that she kissed like Erin Moran (Joanie). "Happy Days" was a popular TV program at the time and from that moment on they lovingly referred to each other as "Joanie and Chachi" a reference to the young love stricken characters in the show.

Not too long afterwards, Mom and Randy were Christmas shopping with their good friends, Guy and Francis Hecker. Guy and Francis loved Randy and many times would take Randy and Gail with them out to dinner and dancing on a double date. Of course Randy and Gail would sit at their own table and play "mooie mooie." Mooie Mooie was Randy and Gail's "secret" code for kissing.

As Mom and Francis did their Christmas shopping, Guy and Randy visited almost every jewelry store in the mall. They looked at many diamond rings, some extremely expensive. They settled on a ¼ karat cubic zirconium, set in a gold band.

A few nights later, Guy and Francis took Randy and Gail to dinner. During dessert, Randy got down on one knee and proposed. In a moment reminiscent of their first kiss she said, "I accept."

The subject of their phone conversations from that point on were centered on their wedding plans. More specifically, what kind of food they were going to serve. It was a wonderful dream but sometimes dreams don't come true.

Randy may dream about being married, but in truth, there's no way he could support a wife, much less a family. The old saying, "Be careful what you wish for, you just might get it" rings painfully true in this situation. Randy is very set in his ways. He adheres to his schedule religiously. If there is one word that describes a successful marriage, it's compromise. Let's face facts; the ability to compromise is not a strong point of an eight year old.

But that's ok. This is yet another example of how Randy gets to have the best of both worlds. Where most people have a thriving love affair, then get married and several years later the heat and passion that brought them together has grown into a relationship based on mutual respect and compromise, Randy gets to live perpetually in the throws of the passionate romance.

So Randy and Gail have now been "engaged" for 24 years. They don't talk as much on the phone as they used to. Gail lives in a group home in Pennsylvania and Randy lives with Mom in Shalimar, Florida. They're apart, but still lovingly together.

Randy's Angels from Destin, Florida

If the names, Jill Munroe, Sabrina Duncan, Kelly Garrett, John Bosley and Charlie Townsend ring a bell, then you were probably one of the millions of viewers who tuned in each week to watch the 1970's action adventure TV show, "Charlie's Angels." The show was about an eccentric millionaire named Charlie Townsend who owned a detective agency staffed by three of the most beautiful women in the world whom he referred to as his "Angels." Each week, Charlie would deliver an assignment by speakerphone to the Angels and dramatic crime fighting action would ensue.

The premise of having beautiful women fight crime at one's behest was then and is today superlative fodder for Randy's fantastic imagination.

"I wish I had my OWN Angels," Randy would mumble after each weekly episode. When the show was canceled in 1981, I'd thought I'd heard the last of it, but the show was soon syndicated, so I got to hear it daily. I heard it for nearly 23 years until April 29 1998, and I haven't heard it since thanks to *my* Angel, my wife Angela.

Angela was enamored with Randy from the moment they met. Be it just or not, I have always judged a person's character by their reaction to and ultimately acceptance of Randy. Most people are cordial, few are not. I once asked a young woman I had been casually dating if she was interested in dating more seriously. She told me she could never have a serious relationship with me because ultimately she thought there would be an increased chance us having a child with Down Syndrome. I wondered if she really believed that or if she was using it as an excuse to get out of dating me. In either case, she showed her true character and I showed myself to the door.

Angela was different. Not long after we started dating, she made a date with Randy to go to lunch and a movie. I wasn't invited. It was just Angela and Randy. Randy's face gleamed with pride when she arrived to pick him up for their date.

"Don't worry brother, I'll take good care of her," he said with a Cheshire cat grin as he climbed into her car.

As they drove away, it occurred to me that Angela was taking Randy on a "Buddy Buddy" day like I had done so many times. She genuinely enjoyed his company. She showed her true character and a few months later I, on bended knee, showed her a ring.

So on April 29 1998, Randy's wish came true. Angela along with our friends Kathy, Susan and Kimberlee gave him a T-shirt with their pictures on it with the caption "Randy's Angels." By the look on his face you would have thought they had just given him a winning lottery ticket. That T-shirt is one of his most prized possessions, alongside his TV Guide collection and Dad's comb.

They also came up with an idea for Randy to give them an assignment which they would carry out and report back to him. The assignment Randy came up with was for the *Angels* to go on a Disney Cruise and submit a written report of their experiences upon their return.

Randy has been on several cruises and he loves them. He especially loves the fact that on a cruise you can eat to your hearts content at any time of the day or night. He also loves anything Disney. So it's not hard to understand why he would combine the two for his Angel's assignment. The thought of his *Angels* on a cruise ship with Disney characters was just euphoric.

Of course the *Angels'* work schedules and the costs made it impractical for them to actually go on this cruise assignment but that wasn't important. What *was* important was that Randy got to imagine it all happening!

For months, Randy would call each of them and ask them how their assignment was coming along. They all played along and told him all the characters they met and all the food they were having. He knew they weren't actually on the cruise but he was pretending to be Charlie and *that* was fun. The phone calls became part of his daily routine almost to the point of being obsessive. The *Angels* never complained, but Mom noticed this and suggested he limit his calls to once or twice a week, which Randy agreed.

A little less than a year later, the *Angels* organized a party where they would present the final report of their assignment. They cut and pasted pictures of themselves and Disney characters from cruise brochures and placed them along with a creative written narrative of their adventure into a three ring binder. At the party they presented the report along with a new Randy's Angels T-Shirt because he had practically worn out the first shirt they gave him. He cherishes that report and has it displayed in a place of prominence on his desk to this day.

While Randy certainly loves having his very own *Angels,* being one of Randy's Angels has become a desirable position. Several of our friends have wanted to join the *Angels* but Randy has stood faithful to his core group with one exception, our friend Karen. Karen's initial request for admission was denied but she was persistent and finally got Randy to agree to let her become an *Angel,* but there were conditions. First she had to get the approval of the other Angels, which wasn't easy. Second, the *Angels* had to create a new T-shirt that included Karen. Lastly, she had to participate in an induction ceremony. The stage was set for another party.

At the party, Randy and his *Angels* sequestered themselves in his den for the top secret induction ceremony. I wish I could have video taped it but Randy made it clear that no one else at the party was allowed in the room with them. Behind the door we could hear them laughing. Five minutes later they emerged looking like they had just come from a comedy club. Angela later told me that he started by introducing Karen to her friends of many years. Next he held out a stack of TV Guides and asked her to place her left hand on the stack and raise her right hand. They could hardly contain themselves.

He then said, "Repeat after me. I, Karen, pledge allegiance to Randy and to be the best Angel I can be. So help me Randy"

And it was done.

The Angels still get together periodically for an Angel's party where they usually give Randy a new T-Shirt. He has about nine of them now and he proudly wears them all.

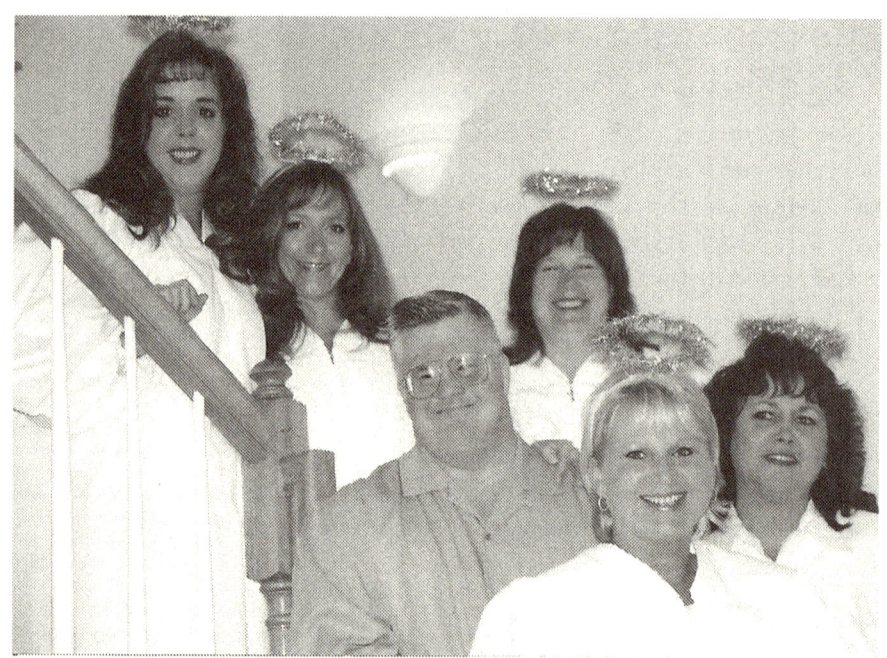

Randy's Angels

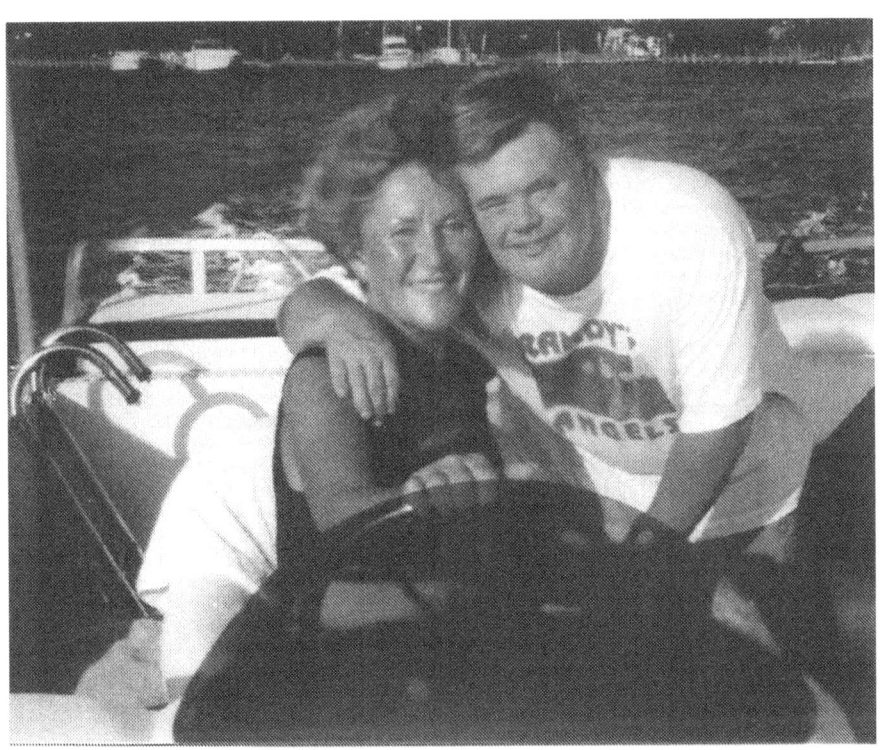

Randy and Mom

10

The Heart of Down Syndrome

"Love to faults is always blind, always is to joy inclin'd, lawless, wing'd, and unconfined and breaks all chains from every mind."—William Blake

The Sara Bonwell Hudgins Center (SBHC) in Hampton, Virginia is a remarkable place. It was founded in 1967 as a non-profit organization dedicated to enhancing the lives of people with mental and/or physical disabilities. It has a 38-acre campus that includes residences, a vocational/industrial center, a gymnasium and a state-of-the art child development center. Many people with Down Syndrome and other disabilities lived and/or worked there; others, like Gooma, lived with their families but went to the center to either work or play. They held lots of social events that Gooma loved to attend including, sock-hop dances, cook outs, bowling tournaments, and Special Olympics.

When I was sixteen years old, I drove Gooma to a birthday party for a friend of his at SBHC. Usually I would have stayed for the party but I had something else to do that day so I stopped in and briefly greeted and hugged some of the partygoers, many of whom I knew from other SBHC events, then left. When I picked him up a few hours later I asked him how the party was and if he had fun. He said he had a great time and that he met a new friend named "Matt" who he thought was really funny.

"Who was Matt?" I asked.

Gooma had a hard time describing Matt to me. His first observation was that Matt was the one who had *two* pieces of cake. I asked him what Matt was wearing.

Randy replied, "You know, the usual, jeans and a shirt." I asked him what color Matt's shirt was.

He said, "I don't know, blue, I think, or maybe red." I then asked what Matt looked like.

He said, "You know, normal."

This went on for a few more minutes as I quizzed him on Matt's appearance, (height, weight, etc.) to see if I could remember which one at the party was Matt. Each of Gooma's answers were vague and I could sense he was getting frustrated with my insistent questions that he had no "right" answer for so I dropped it.

A couple of weeks later, I took Gooma to another SBHC function. This time I stayed. When we arrived, Gooma was anxious to point Matt out to me. He scanned the crowd until he found him then eagerly led me to him and introduced us. Matt and I shared the traditional "Rand-Shake" as I sometimes called it back then. (At any SBHC function, when you meet someone new, the common greeting isn't a handshake like in most of society, the common greeting is a hug.) We chatted briefly and Matt was indeed charming.

Matt had Down Syndrome and was about 5'5" tall with a stocky build and a bald head. I remembered seeing Matt at the birthday party a couple weeks prior. To me he stood out because Matt was the only African American person at the party. When Gooma didn't immediately say to me that Matt was the "black" guy, I crossed him off my mental list of potential people as Gooma's new friend. Gooma never saw Matt as black. He didn't even see Matt as bald. He saw Matt for who he really was; a charming, friendly, funny, loving human being.

I never forgot that lesson. Many years later, I had a roommate named Corey. My Mom asked me to tell her about my new roommate so I told her where Corey was from, where he worked, that he was a great guy and that we had a lot in common. She invited us to dinner one night and she just loved him. As we were leaving that night, Mom pulled me aside and whispered, "You didn't tell me Corey was black," I said, "Well, he didn't ask me if you were white." Thanks to my Brother/Humanities teacher, to this day, I never use color to define anyone.

It's important to keep in mind that the "Down" in Down Syndrome was the name of the person for whom the syndrome was named and has nothing to do with their attitudes, demeanor or direction in life. Rex Hudler, the announcer for the California Angels and a very popular former major league baseball player, uses the term "Up" Syndrome to reframe our thinking about the condition.

If we gauge intelligence by one's performance on a test or the depth and breadth of one's vocabulary or one's mathematical or scientific comprehension then by that standard, people with Down Syndrome may fall short. However, if we gauge intelligence by one's grasp of humanity, then they far surpass us all.

When Gooma meets someone, he doesn't care what they do for a living or how much money they make. He doesn't care about politics or what religion they follow. He doesn't care if they are tall or short; fat or thin; old or young; pretty or plain; black or white. He harbors no hatred, jealousy, animosity or prejudice. When Gooma meets someone, he cares about the living beating heart in their chest; a kind smile on their face; and a warm strong embrace. He cares about family and friends, good music and food, laughter and love. He may not have a 140 IQ, but he is an expert at being human.

With patience and love, a family will come to realize that they have been given a great gift. A special child brings a very special love. These children strengthen a family, provide a different perspective on every day life, and are a real joy to be around. Randy has brought great love and joy into our family, and none of us would change him, even if we could.

EPILOGUE:
Chess Match

One day when Gooma was about 20 years old, he had the idea he should receive an allowance. After mulling this over in his head for a while, he gathered the courage to go downstairs and ask Dad. He wasn't very confident of Dad's reaction. His shoulders were tight and approaching his earlobes. His chin planted firmly in his chest. His hands rooted deeply in his pockets. The door to Dad's office was barely cracked open. Gooma poked his head in and saw Dad working at his desk, his back to the door. Dad heard the door creak.

"Hey Bud," Dad said without looking up. "Come on in"

"Are you sure?" Gooma said in his trademark tenuous tone as he entered the office like a kid wading into a cold pool. "I'm not interrupting you am I?"

Dad took his reading glasses off and turned around. He had enjoyed watching Gooma make the same approach many times. He expected Gooma to ask him to go to McDonalds or to read the latest entry in his TV Guide log. Dad knew Gooma well, his patterns, and the way he dealt with his concerns. But every once in a while, Gooma surprised him.

"What can I do for you Son?" Dad said, a gleam in his eye.

Gooma searched for just the right way to say what he had to say. He rubbed his hands nervously as if they were beneath one of those electric hand dryers in a public restroom.

"Umm, Dad?" He began. "Um, I, Um." A long pause followed while Gooma gathered the words. "I, I, I've been thinking. Tell me what you think about this. What would you say if, um."

"What is it Randy?" Dad said to help speed along the process.

"OK, here it goes. I've got an idea." Gooma stalled just a little more. "How about if I get an allowance?"

Whew! He said it. His shoulders dropped, his chin lifted. You could see the relief on his face at just getting the question out.

Without hesitation, Dad said, "I think that's a grand idea Bud."

"You do?" Gooma said, His eyes wide and bright as if he'd just been told he'd won the lottery.

"Absolutely!" Dad said, "You take out the garbage. You clean your room. You unload the dishwasher and you put the flag out every morning and take it in every night. You deserve an allowance."

He was not sure where Gooma got the idea but he knew it had been brewing in his head for some time now. Things like this are not easy for Gooma. It takes time for him to formulate the thought and to express it. Dad always recognized this and was proud that Gooma had done so well.

"How much do you want?"

Gooma's expression changed from that of a kid walking into Disney World to that of a dog tilting its head slightly when it hears a strange noise. He hadn't thought that far ahead. He had spent all that mental energy on the initial question. Now Dad had to throw in a little twist.

"Um. I'll be right back," Gooma said then scurried off to his room to contemplate an amount. Dad chuckled to himself then went back to work. He knew it would be at least ten minutes before Gooma returned. Then as sure as if he had been timing it, Gooma entered the room. He didn't wait for Dad to invite him in. Although ten minutes had passed, Gooma was still in the moment.

"Dad, Um, I've been thinking," Gooma said with much less hesitation. "How about ten dollars?"

"Perfect! Ten dollars it is. You deserve it." "What day do you want to receive your allowance?"

"I'll be right back," Gooma said and headed back to his room to contemplate some more. The nervousness that turned to anticipation had now turned to frustration. You could hear it in his step. The sound of his feet hitting the steps was louder than before.

This exchange had turned into something of a chess match between a master that can anticipate many moves in advance and the novice that must move one piece at a time to decide where to go next.

The stopwatch hit ten minutes and Dad knew it was time for Gooma to make his next move. He heard him coming down the stairs and turned around to greet him. Gooma began right where they left off.

"Dad, how does Friday sound to you?" Gooma said, sounding more like a negotiator now.

"Fantastic," Dad said, "You will get a ten dollar allowance every Friday from now on." Dad now had to put in his final move. "Of course remember, that you have to keep up your chores. If you don't do your chores, then you don't get your allowance. Deal?"

"Deal!" Gooma says

Dad had played this game masterfully. Although Gooma always did do his chores, he now had an incentive and a reward. Dad was good at teaching Gooma.

"Now I've got to get back to work Bud. I'll see you later." Dad said as he put his glasses on and went back to work.

"Ok, thanks Dad," Gooma said as he turned to leave the office.

"You're welcome, Son," Dad said without looking up.

Suddenly Gooma turned back around and said, "Oh yeah, Dad, one more thing."

What is it now? Dad thought. He was a patient man but sometimes he had to put his foot down in order to get anything done. Dad turned around one more time. He was going to tell Gooma to 'run along' so he could get some work done but the ear-to-ear grin on Gooma's face stopped him.

"What is it Bud?"

Gooma held out his hand and said, "Today's Friday!"

Check mate!

ABOUT THE AUTHORS

Robert (Opey) Russ lives in Santa Rosa Beach, Florida, with his wife Angela and their son Jackson. Opey works as a Financial Planner for Brewster Brown Financial Group, Inc. and his wife Angela works as a Speech Pathologist for Fort Walton Medical Center. His email address is opey@opey.com.

Robin Lindenmeier lives in Richland, Washington, with her husband Clark and their two children, Ryan and Sarah. Robin works as a Project Management Specialist for Battelle Northwest National Laboratory and her husband Clark works as a Scientist for Battelle Northwest National Laboratory. Her email address is beana@opey.com.

Jean and Randy (Gooma) Russ live in Shalimar, Florida. Jean is a homemaker and Randy works for Burger King and Albertsons five days per week. They are healthy, happy, busy and enjoying life. Randy is 49 years old. Jean's email address is JeanRuss@Cox.net.

Michael Levin lives in California and works as an author and consultant. In addition to reviewing the manuscript and providing editorial comments and suggestions, Michael coached and inspired us all to find the story within. Thank you Michael!

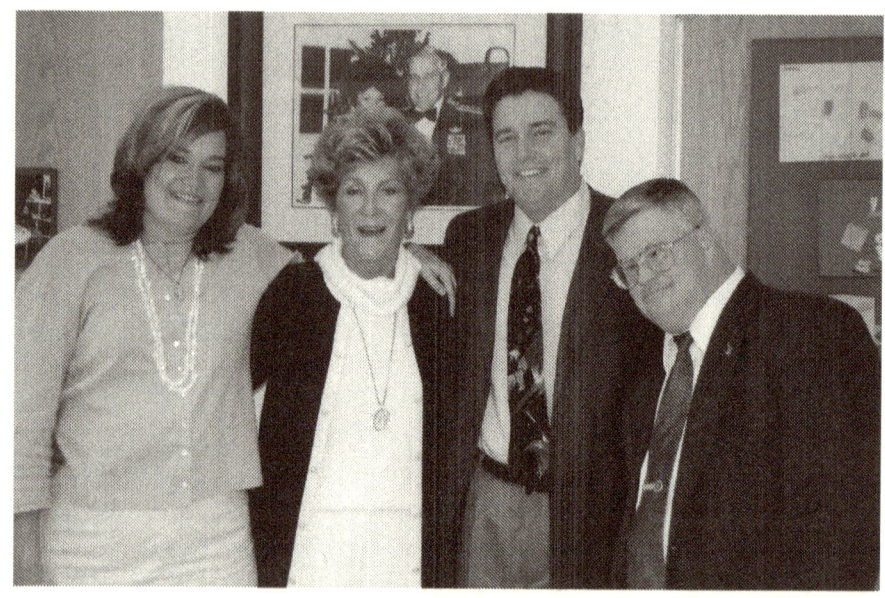

Robin, Mom, Opey, Randy

978-0-595-47367-0
0-595-47367-9